THE SHAPE OF THE HEART

THE SHAPE
OF
THE HEART

BY

PIERRE VINKEN

ELSEVIER

Colophon
Design Anton Ross • Production Henk van Es • Translations Peter Mason
• Lithography Repro de Jong/Studio Ross • DTP Fokker Drukwerk, Amsterdam •
Printing Boom Planeta de Grafische, Haarlem • Printed in The Netherlands
• The paper used in this publication meets the requirements of ANSI/NISO
z39.48-1992 (Permanence of paper). See also page 208.
ISBN: 0-444-82987-3
Reprinted with revisions, January 2000

In the main, the illustrations are either reductions or enlargements of the originals. In many cases only a detail is shown.

WHY IS THE HEART NOT HEART-SHAPED?

A recent CD-ROM disc of an interactive educational programme devoted to the heart and entitled *Smart heart* (fig.1) carried a label featuring a large, red Saint Valentine's heart. But the case in which the disc was presented showed a picture of a real heart. Both illustrations featured the heart, yet they were entirely dissimilar.

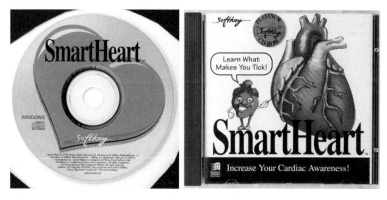

Fig.1. *Smart Heart*, CD-ROM and case, published by Softkey, Wimbledon Common, 1995.

The question of why we are accustomed to depict the heart so differently from its actual shape was raised by the well-known art historian Erwin Panofsky. He wrote: 'The heart has always fascinated me, not only because of the famous controversy about the perforations of the *saeptum* (which Galen postulates, which Leonardo claims to have seen, and which even Vesalius accepts) but also because I could never find out when, where and how the schematization into what we call heart-shaped form ♡ came about. It is already found in one paleolithic cave, and I have never been able to understand the *Gestalt*-psychological process by which the scalloped upper contour came about' (fig.2). Panofsky did not attempt to provide an answer to the question. In this case, the great man was, to quote Aby Warburg, perhaps less interested in a solution than in the formulation of a new problem.

here and how the schema
 form ♡ came about
nd I have never been at
ogical process by which

Fig.2. Fragment from a letter by Erwin Panofsky to the author, dated 17 October 1961.

The elegant, scalloped contour of the Valentine heart is probably the most universal icon in the world. But its shape cannot be derived from observation of an actual heart, because it does not look like one. About 1500, Leonardo da Vinci drew a large number of hearts, seen from the outside and from the inside, apparently on the basis of his own observations (fig.3). They were often the hearts of animals, but the shape of the heart of a monkey, pig or cow is not essentially different from that of a human being. None of the contours of Leonardo's

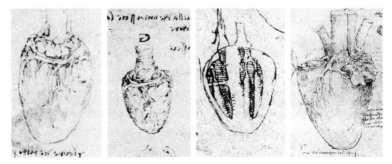

Fig.3. Hearts drawn by Leonardo da Vinci, about 1500.

drawings resembles the small heart icon in Panofsky's letter. A real heart looks like a roughly fist-sized, light brown, cone-shaped clod; anyone who wants to represent a genuine heart knows very well that it cannot be done with the contour of the Valentine heart. If a real heart looks like those of Leonardo, which it does, one may well wonder why we have been representing it in the shape that we see, for example, on playing cards.[1]

Panofsky's question can be expanded upon. A characteristic of some heart images, such as those on playing cards, is that the sides are concave. This is not to be found in real hearts, nor does a real heart have a sharp tip at the bottom, though this may be the unintended result of having given the heart icon concave sides. Surprisingly, Panofsky considered a psychological process to be responsible for the occurrence of the heart icon, a rather unexpected postulate from one of the fathers of iconology.

The shape of the heart has undergone a complex development. Its Greek anatomical history is relatively easy to follow, but varying conceptual differences amongst classical authors led to major confusion in the middle ages. One particular misunderstanding gave rise to the appearance of a dent or fold in the upper side of the heart. The outline of the scalloped heart icon can be found on many occasions since antiquity, but this was never intended to be taken as an illustration of the heart; neither in the middle ages, nor in classical times.

Panofsky's observation that the 'heart-shaped' form is to be found in a paleolithic cave refers to the painting of a red-coloured elephant in the cave of Pindal in Spain (fig.4). The cave was discovered by the French *abbe* Henri Breuil. He made a drawing of the elephant at the site, believing that the mark on the animal's upper body was meant to represent its ear, and it is so described in his 1911 report: 'A large, more or less heart-shaped mark, situated in the middle of the body, represents the ear flap'. It was later suggested to him by elephant hunters that the mark might have been intended to represent the heart rather than the ear, because a painting of another elephant in a later prehistoric cave in Southern France shows it being pierced by three arrows above the left

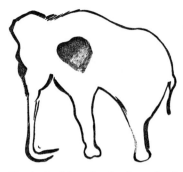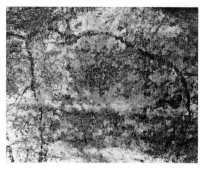

Fig.4. Prehistoric elephant in the cave of Pindal, Spain. Left Breuil's drawing, right his photograph.

shoulder, the spot where the animal could most easily be brought down. Breuil did not reject the suggestion, and whilst he never proposed that the stone age painter had been depicting a heart, he did agree that the mark was approximately where the elephant's heart would be.[2]

Many years later, Richard Lewinsohn discussed the subject in detail with Breuil. He felt that the latter had been too easily swayed by the elephant hunters and that this had led to the subsequent belief that the mark did indeed represent the animal's heart. In Lewinsohn's view, the mark, which Breuil had copied under difficult circumstances in the narrow, dark cave, was oval rather than triangular, with a flat, rather than scalloped, upper side. Indeed, a comparison of the drawing with the actual photograph shows that the patch in the latter lacks a clear contour. It bears no resemblance to the actual shape of the heart, nor does it resemble the mark as copied by Breuil. It is too indistinct even to support Lewinsohn's contention that it has an oval contour.[3]

The oldest known representation of a heart is a 3000-year-old Olmec effigy vessel found in Mexico (fig.5). It is a two-part anthropomorphic ceramic container. The torso has the rough shape of a heart, with three large blood vessels protruding from the rounded base. The belly of the figure seems to consist of two chambers, and the interventricular furrow *(anterior longitudinal sulcus)* is

10

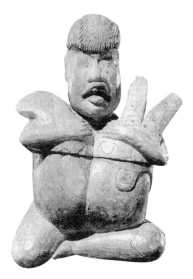

Fig.5. Olmec ceramic heart-shaped effigy vessel, 1200-900 BC.

visible in the outer wall. The vessel may have served as a sacrificial receptacle, perhaps to contain blood, but its true purpose remains unclear. The object is unique, thus making comparative study impossible. We also encounter pictorial or sculptural representations of the heart in other Mesoamerican classical cultures (fig.6), but, of course, these rather realistic heart shapes cannot have had any influence on that given to representations of the heart in Europe before the sixteenth century.[4]

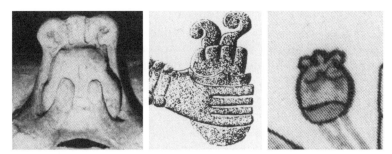

Fig.6. Mayan and Aztec hearts: detail of a ceramic statuette, early classical period; a detail of *Piedra itzpapalotl*, Mexico, and human heart sacrifice by an Aztec priest. Ends of the blood vessels are still attached to the base of the hearts.

An early, Egyptian notion of the shape of the heart is to be found in Plutarch's book on the myth of *Isis and Osiris*. He wrote that the peach-tree was consecrated, in particular, to Isis because its fruit resembles a heart. There are no direct Egyptian sources on its shape. It played an important role as the seat of intelligence and wealth, wisdom and feeling. The ancient Egyptians believed that it was needed in the afterlife, since it would be weighed in the balance at judgement time. But the heart was never depicted, perhaps because of a taboo. It was embalmed separately and put into a canopic jar, which became the representation of the heart (fig.7). Many of these urns, forgetting their lids, look something

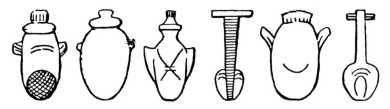

Fig.7. Early Egyptian representations of the heart.

like a real heart. A schematic representation of it passed into the hieroglyphic system as the symbol for 'heart'. Sometimes, the urns had handles, a natural accessory for a pitcher, but they may also have been intended to represent those parts of the heart that are still called heart ears, *auricula*. Later on, probably because improved techniques of mummification enabled the natural heart to be left inside the corpse, the heart urn was replaced by a stone 'heart scarab' which was positioned on the breast of the mummy. These amulets were beetle-shaped, and bore no resemblance to a peach or to the modern heart icon.[5]

The Greek literature on the shape of the heart is rather sparse. None of the classical or medieval anatomists appears to have paid it much attention. We find a few lines on its appearance, followed, usually without any evident transition, by a lengthy text on its supposed functioning. Aristotle describes the shape of the heart in his *History of animals* as follows:

> The heart has three cavities (...). The rounded end of the heart is at the top. The pointed end is very largely fleshy and firm in texture (...) its shape as a whole is not elongated but roundish, except of course that it is pointed at the end. It has three cavities, the largest being on the right hand side, the smallest on the left, and the medium-sized one in the middle.[6]

The Hippocratic corpus, a large collection of writings from the Hippocratic school, most of which dates from the fourth century BC, includes a separate treatise on the heart, probably written in the first half of the third century BC. It too describes the heart as round (rounder than in any other animal) and pyramid-shaped:

> In shape the heart is like a pyramid (...). It is enveloped in a smooth membrane. In this membrane there is a small quantity of fluid, rather like urine, giving one the impression that the heart moves in a kind of bladder (...). It contains in one circumference two separate cavities [chambers], one here, the other there. These cavities are quite dissimilar (...). Furthermore [the right] chamber is very spacious, and much more hollow than the other. It does not extend to the extremity of the heart, but leaves the *apex* solid, being as it were stitched on the outside.[7]

Galen, the second-century Greek physician who studied in Pergamon and Alexandria and later practiced in Rome, summarized the medical knowledge of the ancient world, describing the heart most fully in two different works: in the sixth book of *The usefulness of the parts*, and in the second part of the seventh book of *Anatomical procedures*. He too described the shape of the heart as a cone with the tip pointing downwards:

> ... the heart is not perfectly spherical and (...) beginning at the broad, circular base above, which is called the head, it gradually decreases in size, very like a cone, and becomes narrow and slender at its lower end. [8]

Greek texts were studied, translated and disseminated by the Byzantines and Arabs. Galen's works became the basis of all teaching and investigation until the sixteenth and seventeenth centuries. Much of it, with very little change to the anatomical knowledge, was incorporated in the works of scholars from the tenth and eleventh centuries, such as Rhazes and Haly Abbas, and above all in the *Canon of medicine*, the great Arab compendium by Avicenna, court physician in Hamadan, written around the year 1000. It was translated into Latin in the twelfth century, and together with the work of Galen, it formed the basis of medieval western medicine. The *Canon* describes the shape of the heart as being:

> large, because the arteries originate there. The large part of the heart is on the upper side (...) it has a tapered form and is small at the lower end. (...) The heart contracts to the shape of a pine-cone, so that it assumes the appropriate form above and below and has no redundancy (...). In the heart are three ventricles, two are large, and the third as it were between (...). The heart has two accessory parts (small ears) placed at the two openings through which two materials enter: blood and air. These parts resemble ears, they are wrinkled and flaccid when the heart contracts (...). The heart is turned slightly to the left.[9]

The descriptions by Avicenna's Arab predecessors are similar but shorter. The Persian physician, Rhazes, writes that 'the shape of the heart resembles an inverted pine-cone which from the head is tapered downwards and whose root (base) faces upwards (...) the apex [tip] of the cone is turned to the left (...) the heart has two ventricles (...)'. Haly Abbas wrote more or less the same:

> the shape resembles a pine-cone and its large base faces upwards (...) its conical tip is turned to the left (...). There are two ventricles (...) there is no third ventricle. (...). Each of the heart chambers has two accessory parts on the outside which look like ears and which are called the heart ears.[10]

The descriptions of the outside of the heart by the classical writers were usually brief, but correct and adequate. Its shape held no secrets for them, because from prehistoric times down to the twentieth century, almost everyone must have seen the heart of a dead animal, and people have always (rightly) assumed that the heart of a pig or cow looks like that of a human being.

Johannes Mesue, an eclectic translator and compiler living about 1100, also wrote that the heart has a pine-cone shape and that the upper side of the heart is convex in order to provide sufficient room for the large blood vessels to be able to enter the heart. The great medieval *doctor universalis* Albertus Magnus (1206-1280), drawing his medical knowledge from Arabic-Latin versions of Aristotle and Avicenna, repeats that the heart has the conic shape of a pine-cone. The same can be found in Henri de Mondeville's book of anatomy from 1304 and in the influential *Anathomia* (1316) of his Bolognese colleague and contemporary Mundinus (c.1275-1327). It is stated there that the heart has the shape of a pyramidal pine-cone, a combination of the Hippocratic pyramid and Avicenna's pine-cone. The *Anathomia Mundini* was an important bridge between classical and Arabic anatomy, on the one hand, and early humanist medicine, on the other. It was the most important textbook until the sixteenth century, and it circulated in a large number of manuscripts before eventually being printed. The book certainly saved its author from the oblivion that comes with old age, a wish that – quoting Galen – he expressed in his dedication.[11]

The standard work on surgery of the fourteenth century, *La grande chirurgie* (1363), by Guy de Chauliac, a pupil of Mundinus' successor Bertuccio and a product of the medical schools of Bologna and Mondeville's Montpellier, also describes the shape of the heart as that of an inverted pine-cone with the tip pointing downwards and the 'root' upwards.[12]

The same description is still found two hundred years later in Vesalius and in the works of later authors down to the present day, e.g. in *Gray's anatomy* (1995),which still uses the ancient formulation: the heart is placed obliquely in the thorax, and it is an organ of a somewhat conical or pyramidal form, with a base, apex and a series of surfaces. None of the anatomists since antiquity, of whom an increasing number have seen the human heart, certainly since 1300, has had reason to change the classical description of the external shape of the heart.[13]

It is remarkable that, outside the anatomical context, there are no early medieval illustrations of the heart extant. It is often mentioned in the literature of the middle ages as a symbol of love, both spiritual and worldly. The association of love with the heart, of the heart as the seat of love, attracted renewed interest in the Provençal courtly literature and in the mystic poetry of the German and French monastic writers in the twelfth century. But the heart was not depicted in the early illuminated manuscripts.[14]

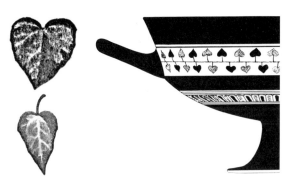

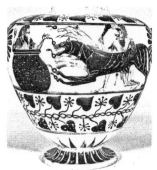

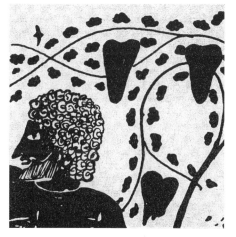

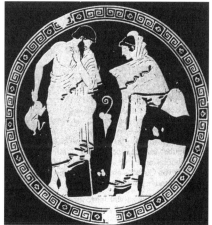

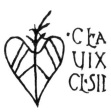

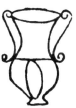

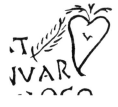

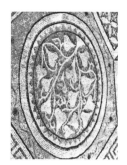

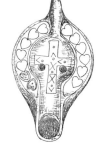

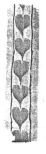

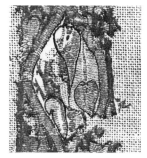

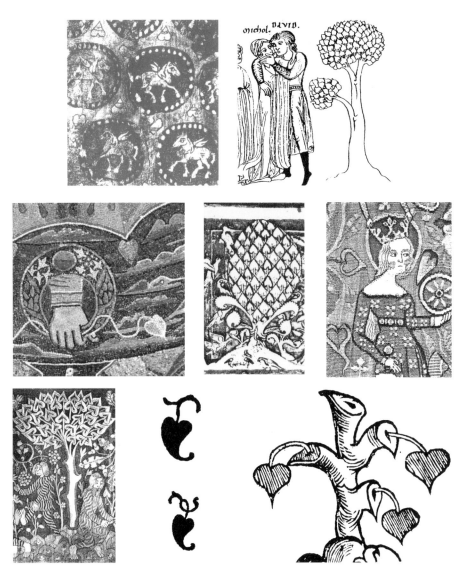

Fig. 8. Page 17: from left to right: photocopied ivy leaves, Siana cup with red and black ivy leaves, 550 BC, hydra from Caere, 550-525 BC, a solitary leaf, or bunch of grapes, on a bowl by Douris, 480 BC, bunches of grapes on a amphora, about 510 BC, ornamental leaves in Roman inscriptions, floor mosaic from Deir shargi, AD 361, North African red ware lamp, 5th century, Coptic textile with red heart-shaped leaves. Page 18: 7th century, heart leaves between *pegasoi* on a Coptic textile, 6th-7th centuries, tree with heart leaves in Petrus Lombardus' *Psalmen Kommentar*, about 1180, leafy figures as Pentecostal tongues in the Omnipotent hand, San Clemente basilica, Rome, 12th century, black and red leaves in *Carmina burana*, about 1230, antependium, about 1400, Regensburg textile, about 1400, leaf ornaments from 16th-century books (see figure 70), printer's mark of Conrad Baumgarten, about 1500.

Figures that resemble the heart icon are common in antiquity, but they do not represent the heart; they are used decoratively, and consist of a bunch of grapes or (ivy) leaves, sometimes with tendrils. These leaves are often depicted with a stalk, which makes them look like the suit of spades in playing cards. Archaeologists refer to this ornamental leaf as the *folium hederae*, spade leaf, or ivy. It also occurs regularly as a graphic decoration in Roman inscriptions in stone or applied to the walls of catacombs. After the Roman era and through the late middle ages we find ivy leaves in ornaments in Byzantine art and in Western Europe. Heart-shaped leaves also occur in Coptic textiles, in representations of Bacchic revels and as a herbal remedy in medieval medical texts. From the renaissance onwards, we find ivy leaves being used as decorative elements in printed books (fig.8).[15]

It has been claimed that a heart is depicted on a fragment of a Roman pot from the Augustan period (fig.9). The surface of this heart would then be roughly four times the size of that of a hand, i.e. more than four times larger than its actual size. In fact, the priest

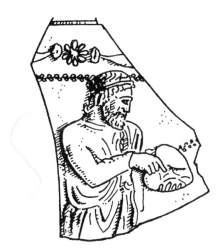

Fig.9. Terra sigillata fragment with a *haruspex* viewing a liver, Augustan period.

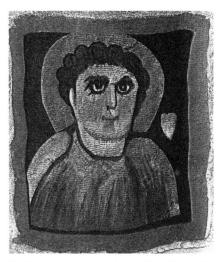

Fig.10. Portrait, Coptic textile, about 400.

portrayed on this fragment is a *haruspex* inspecting entrails, and the organ is not a heart but a liver.[16]

Certain scholars have suggested that a heart is illustrated on a Coptic textile from the fourth or fifth century (fig.10). A small but conspicuous reddish spot features in the background of this portrait, which is woven in early Byzantine style. It is shaped like a long, tapering pear with a dip in the upper side. Others have observed that, in view of the aureole surrounding the head of the figure portrayed, the portrait must be of a Greek god or Christian saint who has a heart as an attribute. Another view is that it represents the prophet Ezekiel, who wrote that God's word would 'take away the stony heart out of your flesh, and [...] give you a heart of flesh'. It has also been suggested that it is a portrait of the Emperor Constantine, or Saint Augustine, who, in the late middle ages, was represented with a heart. There are no grounds to support any of these hypotheses.[17]

There is also no reason for assuming that the artist was seeking to represent a heart. The elongated, scalloped form with its strongly tapering lower end cannot have been based on direct observation of a heart. Nor could it have been derived from the existing descriptions of the heart, although it is somewhat reminiscent of Galen's statement that the heart becomes narrow and slender at its lower end. However, it does not have the roundish shape which, as Aristotle explicitly stated, is not elongated. Nor does it have the 'broad, circular base above' of Galen, 'rounder than that of any other animal', nor Plutarch's shape of a peach. If the weaver had indeed intended to represent a heart, it would undoubtedly have had the classical Greek shape conventional at the time: rounder and less elongated, with the wide rounded surface at the top, and ending in a cone shape.[18]

The roundish form is confirmed about AD 400 by a Roman contemporary, the *vir clarissimus et illustris* Macrobius, probably also of North African origin, at about the same time as the creation of this Coptic portrait. He writes that 'free-born boys were allowed to wear the heart-shaped figure of the bladder (*bulla*) on the breast, in order that the sight of this figure might remind them that excellence of heart was needed to make them men'.[19]

The bladder-like shape of the heart recalls Hippocrates' description of the heart 'that moves in a kind of bladder'. It also appears as a bladder, or as a large egg, in ceramic models of the internal organs, the so-called polyvisceral ex-voto from the Etruscan era (fig.11). Bladder-shaped hearts were also represented in antiquity as a separate ex-voto, a prayer to a god to be healed or offered to him in thanksgiving. It is tempting to see the enigmatic round contours roughly carved into the left-hand side of the Olmec effigy vessel in figure 5 on page 11 as the projection of a bladder-shaped heart.[20]

The feature in the background of the Coptic textile could perhaps be taken to represent a discoloured leaf or a bunch of grapes, like that shown on a bowl dating from 480 BC or on an amphora from 510 BC (fig.8 on page 17), and in that case, to be a representation of one of the seasons (autumn). Alternatively, it could be Dionysos or

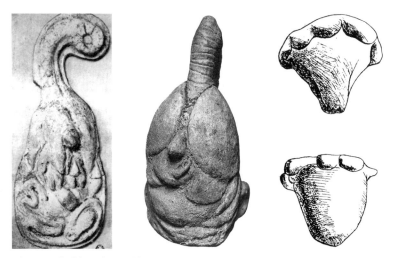

Fig.11. Bladder-shaped hearts as part of Etruscan polyvisceral ex-voto. The hearts appear as egg-shaped bladders between the lung lobes. Right: ceramic Etruscan ex-voto of the isolated heart.

Bacchus, who regularly featured on Coptic textiles accompanied by a nimbus (fig.12). That it should be a bunch of grapes is unlikely, however, since the characteristic setting of leaves and vines is absent.[21]

If the weaver of the portrait had indeed intended the red mark to stand for a human organ, it is more likely to be a tongue than a peach-shaped or pine-cone-shaped heart. Let us consider the complete passage from Plutarch:

> Harpocrates is not to be regarded as an imperfect and an infant god, nor some deity or other that

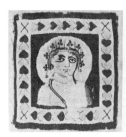
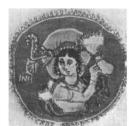
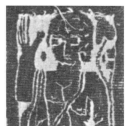

Fig.12. Coptic textiles with *Dionysos*, *Spring* and a dancer, 5th and 6th centuries.

protects legumes, but as the representative and corrector of unseasoned, imperfect, and inarticulate reasoning about the gods among mankind. For this reason he keeps his finger on his lips in token of restrained speech or silence. In the month of Mesore they bring to him an offering of legumes and say, 'The tongue is luck, the tongue is god.' Of the plants in Egypt they say that the *persea* is especially consecrated to the goddess because its fruit resembles a heart and its leaf a tongue. The fact is that nothing of man's usual possessions is more divine than reasoning, especially reasoning about the gods; and nothing has a greater influence toward happiness.[22]

In this passage, the heart is only mentioned incidentally. The focus of attention is the tongue, which is compared to a peach leaf, as a symbol of a wise 'theology', the precondition of human happiness. The red feature in the Coptic portrait looks much more like the pointed leaf of a peach tree than like its fruit. The contour of the scalloped base of the leaf is similar to the base of the human tongue (fig.13). It could perhaps be a

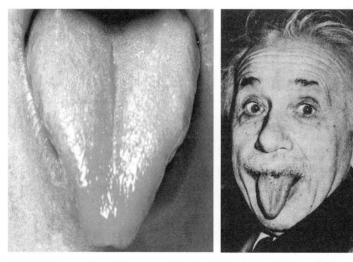

Fig.13. Tongue from the cover of the book *Sensation*, 1997, and the tongue of Albert Einstein.

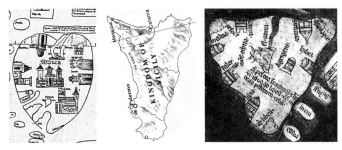

Fig.14. The 'heart-shaped' island of Sicily on the Ebstorf world map (13th century), outline of Sicily from a modern atlas, and Sicily in the Hereford world map, 13th century. The eastern coast of the island faces upward.

representation of Harpocrates, a later version of the ancient Egyptian deity, Horus. Harpocrates was originally the god of Divine reasoning, but in the Graeco-Roman period, he was popularly seen as the god of (wise) silence. Bearing this in mind, we may conclude that this Coptic 'heart' has as little resemblance to an actual heart (or to the shape of the heart as it was known and described at the time) as that on abbe Breuil's paleolithic elephant.[23]

There is another, medieval representation with the form of the heart icon that is just as isolated in its appearance in time as the Coptic heart icon; it is that of the island of Sicily on the famous world map in the monastery of Ebstorf in Germany, dating from the first half of the thirteenth century (fig.14). Scholars have suggested that the island on this map has been given the shape of a heart. The inventor of the map, in all probability the provost of the monastery, Gervase of Tilbury, is supposed to have adopted this shape for Sicily for sentimental reasons because he had been attached to the court there for a number of years. The contour of the island on the Ebstorf world map certainly does resemble a peach, but one from which a couple of bites have been taken on the lower left side.[24]

The exact shape of Sicily was not known in the middle ages. The island (and the other islands in the Medi-terranean) was shown on maps with a variety of outlines:

sometimes as a triangle (a distant relative of its actual shape), but often with another abstract shape, such as a circle, square, rectangle or lozenge. On the Ebstorf map, the island is featured with the eastern coast to the top, and it is scalloped, just as the coast between Messina and Syracuse. Two rivers flow into the bay on the map; two of the several rivers that run into the Gulf of Catania. The bites in the north-western coastline, on the map below left, correspond to the Gulf of Termini Imerese, the Gulf of Castellammare, and a few smaller bays near Palermo. In short, Sicily is here represented more accurately than many other European details on the map, and more accurately than on any other medieval map, including later ones. It is clear that it was drawn by someone who knew the island well.

Sicily is less accurately portrayed on the (later) thirteenth-century Hereford world map, but here too its triangular shape is broken by a dip – deeper than the one on the Ebstorf map – in the middle of the eastern coast. The bays on the north-western coast are also indicated on the Hereford map, but Gervase must have seen them for himself during his stay in Palermo. We may therefore suppose that the scalloped shape of the eastern coast on both maps, and the bays near Palermo on the Ebstorf map, are intended to represent reality. No specific significance can be attached to the rounded outline of the island; Gervase, or whoever drew the map, could not have known whether the northern and southern coasts of the island, each some 360 kilometers long, when seen from the air, were straight, concave or convex. There is thus no need to assume a symbolic 'heart shape' for the island on the Ebstorf map.[25]

Should one persist in maintaining that it had been the cartographer's deliberate intention to feature the island as having the shape of a heart, one would have to explain why, without precedent, he derived the peach-shaped contour of the heart from Plutarch's text. [26]

The earliest known European representations of the heart are perhaps the small silver gilt boxes which were produced in large numbers in eleventh-century Spain (fig.15). But the oldest extant picture since Roman times which can be said with certainty to represent a heart is to be found on an 'anatomical' diagram in an eleventh-century manuscript on which each of the four principal human organs is associated with two of the primary

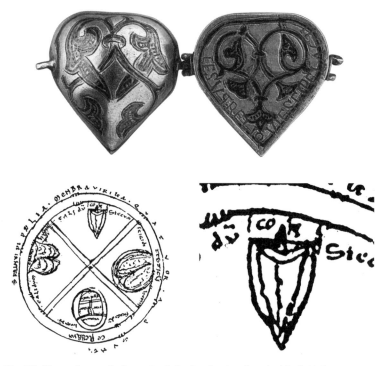

Fig.15. Top: silver gilt box, Andalusia, Spain, first half of 11th century. Below: the oldest known diagram of the heart, from a Cambridge manuscript, about 1100, and detail.

qualities corresponding to the four elements. The heart is characterised by the words 'hot and dry', the pair of qualities that was combined with the element fire, a view which had been foreshadowed by Pythagoras, formulated by Empedocles, and developed by Aristotle; and which became a commonplace after Galen, when it was associated with the heart. The triangular aspect of this heart is meant to reflect on its pyramidal or pine-cone shape. Charles Singer, who reproduced the circular diagram in his chapter on the translators of anatomical texts from the Arabic, called it one of the most childish misrepresentations of ancient doctrines. But as we shall see, this small cross-section actually provides a more accurate picture than any other known sketch of the heart down to the end of the fifteenth century.[27]

The sketch is certainly more accurate than a thirteenth-century illustration on which the signs of the zodiac are connected with the bodily organs. In the centre of the chest is a small imaginary figure that, given its localization and the point in its centre, must be intended to represent the heart. The four-lobed contour does not correspond to any description or illustration of the heart. A circulation man from a very primitive fourteenth-century five-picture series has a similar four-lobed heart (fig.16).[28]

Anatomical sketches of organs must have been current in antiquity as study material as early as the Babylonian and Egyptian cultures. Alexandrian texts written in Greek and provided with didactic schematic

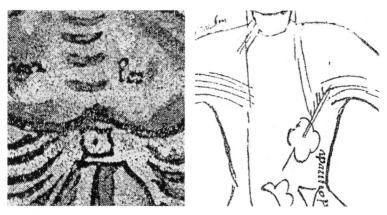

Fig.16. The hearts of an anatomical zodiac figure, 13th century, and of a Circulation man, 14th century.

drawings, probably passed via the medical school of Salerno into medieval European medicine, but none of these classical pictures has survived. Besides plates with sketches of separate organs, which were in use by medieval scholars, surgeons and students, there were sets of primitive anatomical sheets depicting the whole human body, usually in squatting positions. These atlases, which sometimes betray oriental influences, usually consisted of five sheets – hence the name *five-picture series* – in which the osseous, nervous, muscular, venous and arterial systems were represented. None of these sketches was based on actual dissections or original observations.

The oldest known example of such a series is a part of the *Glossarium Salomonis*, a Bavarian manuscript compilation of Latin texts, copied in 1158, in the Pruefening cloister near Regensburg. The heart of the 'circulation man' in this manuscript has the shape of a pine-cone and its apex points to the left (fig.17). There are quite a number of similar series, found all over Europe down to the end of the fifteenth century, all depicting a pine-cone-shaped heart.[29]

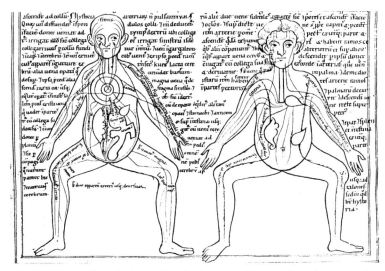

Fig.17. The earliest known Circulation men from a five-picture series, 1158, Pruefening cloister near Regensburg. Left the Vein man, right the Artery man.

Similar sketches can also be seen on a leaf with sketches of organs dating from about 1200, and on an Italian anatomical sheet from the mid-thirteenth century, now in Pisa (fig.18). One of the latter is labelled

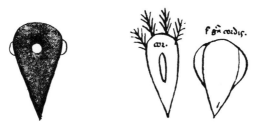

Fig.18. Heart sketch in Codex Caius, about 1200, and two heart diagrams from a Pisan manuscript, 13th century. One of these shows the tree-shaped vessels which spring out of the heart (Galen). The others show the heart-ears.

cor; and from its base emerges the Galenic 'arterial tree', here indicated by four multiple shoots. The second, *figura cordis*, is, like the first of these hearts, drawn with two auricula. The ears also occur in a number of the five-picture series, especially in those showing a Persian influence (fig.19).[30]

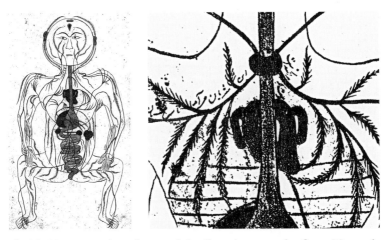

Fig.19. Heart-ears in a figure of the five-picture series from Mansur's *Anatomy*, about 1400, and detail.

The ears were described by Hippocrates, and later by Galen, as *ota*: 'they are thus called from their resemblance to ears, for they grow on either side of the heart as ears on the head'. These ears are, in reality, the external wall of the two *atria*, which form the entrance halls of the main vessels leading into the two larger chambers of the heart. No one knew exactly how to represent them. Because their position and shape had never been accurately described and their function was unclear, they were illustrated in various ways or were simply omitted. They are often mentioned in the medieval anatomical texts, including those by Avicenna, Albertus Magnus, Mundinus, Mondeville and Chauliac. As late as the sixteenth century, we find a pair of shapeless auricles, apparently still not based on observation, attached to a pine-cone-shaped heart in an illustration included in what has been described as the ugliest anatomical work ever published, that by the Parisian anatomist Charles Estienne (fig.20). The shape of the ears, *ridees et laches* (wrinkled and limp), corresponds to the French translation of Avicenna's description.[31]

A noteworthy detail in the early illustrations is the spot that can be seen in the middle of the heart on most

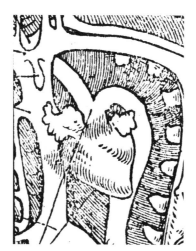

Fig.20. The heart according to Charles Estienne, first half of 16th century. It clearly shows the *sulcus* in the anterior wall and the larger right ventricle.

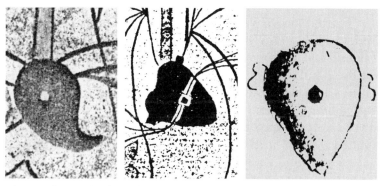

Fig.21. The spot in the middle of the hearts of Circulation men from five-picture series: Caius heart, early 13th century, Raudnitz heart, late 14th century, and an isolated heart sketch from about 1420.

medieval anatomical plates (fig.21). It has been suggested that it stands for the mustard seed mentioned in Mark 4:31, which originates in the heart. But it is not clear why this biblical detail should have been included in an anatomical sketch. One could suggest that it represents the *os cordis,* the heart bone, which was described by classical and medieval anatomists, but is not to be found in the hearts of either humans, pigs, cows or monkeys - the animals most commonly used in dissection. The illuminators did not know what to make of it, and in illustrating obscure texts on the *os cordis,* they could have taken refuge in reproducing this abstract pit in the middle of the pine-cone. However, the fact that the heart bone was situated not in the middle, but at the base of the heart in all the anatomical sources militates against this supposition.[32]

The detailed text accompanying the Raudnitz heart, a relatively late (end of the fourteenth century) version of the five-picture series, provides the key. One of the two plates showing the circulation of the blood contains a heart with not a round, but a square core, which the Latin text describes as a black grain inside the heart (*nigrum granum quod est intus in corde*), in which 'the spirit' resides. The core was thus intended to indicate the place in the heart of the spirit or *pneuma,* the source of its innate heat, and of the pneumatisation of the blood with vital force by which the body is governed.[33]

31

The Galenic 'innate heat' as an essential element in the production of vital spirit is a conception that dates back to the writings of Hippocrates, Plato and Aristotle; it was regarded by scholars in the middle ages as the main function of the heart. The 'circulation figures' of the five-picture series usually occur in pairs, one for the arteries and one for the veins (fig.17 on page 28). As a rule, one of them usually has a heart with a central core, and in the other figure of the pair the position of the heart is often indicated by a (blue) circle or a set of concentric circles, the 'pneuma circle', which indicates that the spirit is driven from the heart by the pulse with the blood to every part of the body.[34]

A less common shape of the heart, mainly in primitive anatomical sketches, is the hazelnut heart, in which the pine-cone heart is represented with disproportionately small lung-lobes (which are sometimes absent altogether) which cover it like a cap over the base, but which do not reach much further than the green ring of small leaves over the base of a hazelnut (fig.22). The source of this negligible role of the lung is an (anatomically not incorrect) observation by Hippocrates that was misunderstood by medieval scholars, who had obviously never seen the relevant organ with their own eyes and

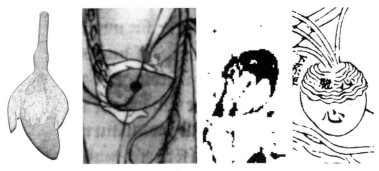

Fig.22. Hazelnut hearts. The first two are taken from a manuscript from 1292, the third is from a Blood-letting man from the second half of the 15th century, the fourth, a Chinese sketch, is from 1692. In the second picture, the windpipe or trachea grips the heart with a miniature lung, like a hand.

who thus represented it incorrectly. Hippocrates writes that the heart is 'enwrapped and cushioned in the lungs, and being surrounded by it'. In fact, the lung is many times larger than the heart, and when viewed from the front, the latter disappears largely behind and between the lobes of the much larger lung as if it were more or less absorbed by it.[35]

THE HEART IN THE VISUAL ARTS

It appears that the first illustration of a heart in Europe outside the anatomical literature occurred in a thirteenth-century French manuscript of the *Roman de la poire* (Romance of the pear), which derives its title from a scene in the story when the damsel offers a pear, analogous to Eve's apple, to her sweetheart. This poem, one of the earliest known Gothic picture cycles devoted exclusively to *fins amours*, has been called a 'Psalter of Love', because its visual structure is modelled on manuscripts of the Psalms. In the *Roman de la poire*, the suitor's gaze is an actual character, Douz Regart (Sweet looks). Within the curve of a golden capital 'S', he is pictured kneeling before the lady and offering her the lover's heart (fig. 23). The text of the *Roman de la poire* dates from circa 1250 and was written by an unknown poet; albeit the name Tibaut, in a reversed anagram, is

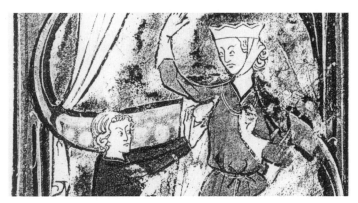

Fig 23. Sweet looks offering the lover's heart, about 1255.

contained in the text. The illustrations were painted in a Paris studio during the period 1250-60. There is a second, markedly similar representation in a later section of the text, viz. the miniature within a capital 'M'. This shows a woman offering a lover's heart to her beau. These are realistic representations of the heart, such as was the case with the Aztecs, and they display the pine-cone form derived from the conventional anatomical texts and illustrations. The same gesture of offering the heart later occurs in the 'public' visual arts, the first such example being that of one of the female figures which Giotto di Bondone painted about 1305 in the Arena chapel in Padua (fig.24). It is Caritas or Divine love offering her heart to God, who appears in the upper right corner. The theme of the surrendering of the heart to God had been described in earlier theological literature, but here it appears for the first time as a visual religious symbol of love. Like its courtly French predecessor, also Giotto's Caritas holds her heart upside down, i.e. at the base; its tip points upwards, very much as an Aztec priest offers a heart to the Sun god (fig.24) and later in a fourteenth-century French ivory (fig. 37 on page 43).[36]

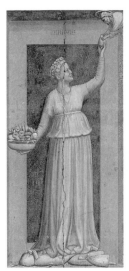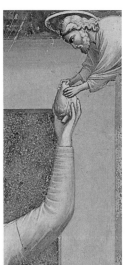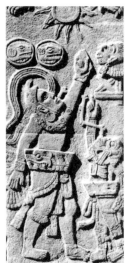

Fig.24. Giotto, *Caritas*, about 1305, Arena chapel, Padua, and detail. Right: Aztec priest offering a human sacrifice heart to the sun.

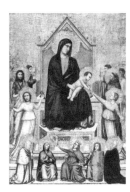 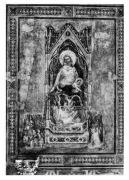 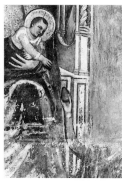

Fig.25. *Madonna with Caritas* by the Master of the Stephaneschi altar, early 14th century, and *Madonna with Caritas*, mural in the Bargello museum, Florence, and detail.

The way in which Giotto's Caritas is offering her heart was immediately picked up by Northern Italian artists. Freyhan mentions a number of similar hearts from the first half of the fourteenth century. From the school of Giotto, we also have a Caritas on a small panel (fig.25). Here Caritas is offering her heart, not to God the Father but to the Child Jesus. Meiss considered this a unique representation: 'nowhere else is the Caritas group merged with the Madonna'. However, there is a virtually identical representation in a badly damaged mural in the Bargello museum in Florence, no doubt from the school of Giotto as well. Here too Caritas offers her heart with her outstretched arm to the Child Jesus, seated on the lap of the Madonna.[37]

Half a mile away from the Bargello is Andrea Pisano's Caritas on the bronze door of the south porch of the Baptisterium, dating from the 1330s. She offers an unscalloped heart, not with her arm outstreched, but rather holding it as an attribute. The latter pose had occurred much earlier, but then a vase was being held (fig.26). It also occurs in a less pronounced form in Giotto's *Allegory of poverty* in the lower church of San Francesco in Assisi, painted between 1330 and 1340 by a follower of Giotto (fig.27).[38]

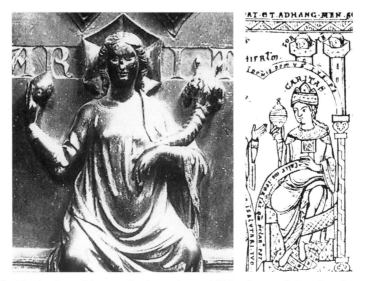

Fig.26. Andrea Pisano, *Caritas*, about 1337, door of Baptisterium, Florence, and *Caritas* from the Ratisbon manuscript, 1165.

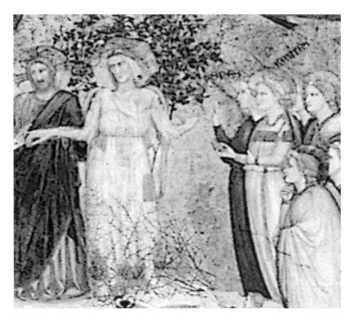

Fig.27. Giotto's *Caritas* offering her heart to Poverty, about 1323, lower basilica of San Francesco, Assisi. Caritas is the figure in white on the right.

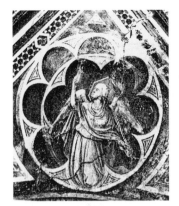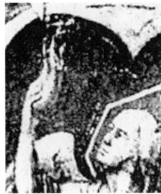

Fig.28. Taddeo Gaddi's *Caritas* with a flame in her hand, about 1330, Santa Croce, Florence, and detail.

About the same time, Taddeo Gaddi painted a Caritas in the Baroncelli chapel of the Santa Croce basilica in Florence. She is not holding a heart, but a flame in her raised hand (fig.28). The association of a Caritas figure with fire or flames in the visual arts dates from the middle of the thirteenth century, when the sculptor Niccola Pisano included on the pulpit of the cathedral in Siena a Caritas figure with a cornucopia from which flames were issuing. Here, the flame symbolizes the fundamental element of Caritas; the fire *(ignis caritatis)* is also burning with cruciform flames behind the head of Giotto's Caritas in Padua (fig.24 on page 34).[39]

The Caritas in the fresco in the Palazzo pubblico in Siena, painted by Ambrogio Lorenzetti about 1340, also holds her heart aloft in her left hand (fig.29). Its flaming point is held upwards. A few years earlier, Lorenzetti had already painted an almost identical Caritas sitting at the feet of the Holy Mother enthroned, holding a long arrow in one hand and a flaming heart in the other. Lorenzetti indicated the names of his Caritas figures in large letters, perhaps to avoid misunderstanding. Nowhere else was the similarity with the Amor figure current in the thirteenth century as great as it was here: a winged, adult Amor, wearing a crown and holding a long arrow, with or without a torch. Caritas' flaming heart also emanates

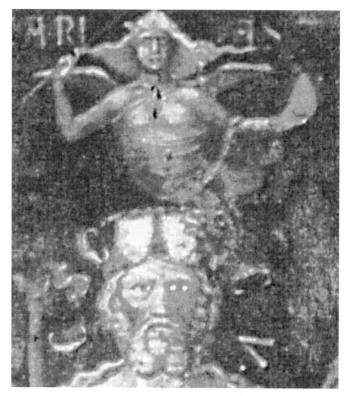

Fig.29. Ambrogio Lorenzetti, *Caritas* with a heart, about 1340, Palazzo Pubblico, Siena.

from Caritas' flaming vessel; as early as circa 1273, Giovanni Pisano sculptured a Caritas with a flaming vase as a caryatid beneath the font in the San Giovanni Fuorcivitas in Pistoia (fig.30). [40]

A Caritas figure, holding a heart as well as a flame, can be found in a mural by Andrea di Bonaiuto on the west wall of the Spanish chapel of the Santa Maria Novella in Florence, painted about 1365 (fig.31). It is one of the three theological virtues above the central figure of Thomas Aquinas. It was assumed that the Caritas figure 'burns with all her flames', referring not only to the flames above her head, but also to those in her hands. Although these small details are no longer clearly visible, we must assume that this Caritas is holding not a flame

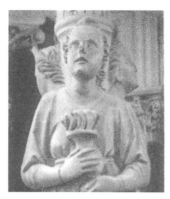

Fig.30. Giovanni Pisano, *Caritas* with flaming vase, about 1272.

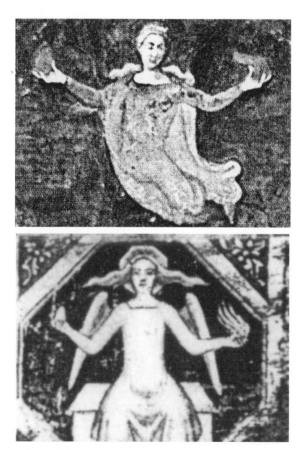

Fig.31. Andrea di Bonaiuto, *Caritas* above Thomas Aquinas and *Caritas* among the Virtues, about 1365, Santa Maria Novella, Florence.

but a heart in her hand – the right hand this time – like the other Caritas figures in Florence, Siena, Padua and Assisi. The red mark in her left hand is larger than the heart in her right hand and its contours are less clear, but it is evident that this hand holds the flame of love. Evidence for this interpretation can be found in the same church; the Spanish chapel contains a second, very similar Caritas figure by the same painter. She is seated among the Virtues, and she too holds a pine-cone heart aloft in her right hand and a flame in her left (fig.31).[41]

Taddeo Gaddi had painted a second Caritas with a conical, flaming heart about 1335, also in the Santa Croce (fig.32). In this case, the heart is as large as a head, so that it has to be lifted with two hands. It may have been the model for the overlarge, flaming hearts of the Caritas by Giovanni di Balduccio (fig.33), and by Andrea Orcagna (fig.34). Much later, in the middle of the fifteenth century, strikingly large hearts, like the Gaddi heart, still recur in the miniatures of the manuscripts of Rene of Anjou (fig.35). One of the sources for the extraordinary size of these hearts may have been the widely known anatomy book by Mundinus, in which it is stated that the human heart is larger than that of any comparable living creature, an exaggeration of a notion deriving from Aristotle. But the painters may also have been directly or

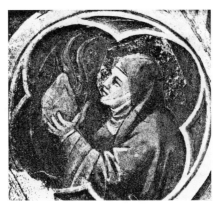

Fig.32. Taddeo Gaddi, *Caritas* with an overlarge flaming heart, about 1335.

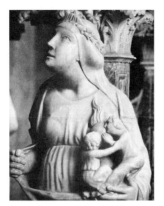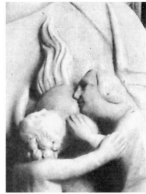

Fig.33. Giovanni di Balduccio, *Caritas*, about 1337, arca of Saint Peter martyr, in S. Eustorgio, Milan, and detail.

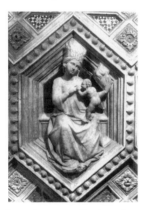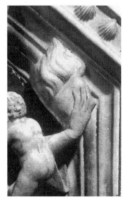

Fig.34. Andrea Orcagna, *Caritas*, about 1357, tabernacle in Orsanmichele, Florence, and detail.

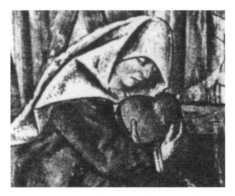

Fig.35. Detail of a miniature from *Le mortifiement de vaine plaisance*, mid-15th century.

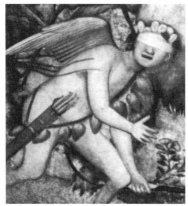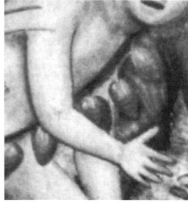

Fig.36. Giotto's *Amor*, about 1323, lower church of San Francesco, Assisi, and detail.

indirectly inspired by a passage from Saint Augustine according to which the heart is enlarged by love for God (*latitudo cordis, quam charitas fecit*).[42]

The pine-cone heart is also found in the art of this period outside the sphere of Caritas, namely in the Allegory of chastity, generally dated about 1323, in the lower church of the basilica of San Francesco in Assisi (fig.36). Panofsky describes the Amor depicted there as a boy of twelve or thirteen who is 'entirely nude, except for the string of his quiver, on which are threaded the hearts of his victims like scalps on the belt of an Indian'.[43]

A later secular example, belonging to the French courtly tradition, is the pine-cone-shaped heart on an ivory object from the first half of the fourteenth century, for example in a courtly scene in which the man kneels and offers his heart up to his beloved not with his hands, but with his cloth (fig.37). The shape of the heart and the gesture with which he offers it to his lady by holding it aloft, may have been derived from earlier French sources (such as the one in figure 23 on page 33), or from Giotto and his Northern Italian followers.[44]

Generally speaking, from the thirteenth century onwards, the heart, whether burning or not, is held by the

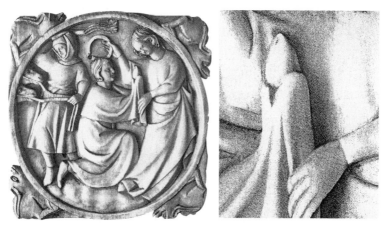

Fig.37. Lover offers his heart to his beloved, ivory mirror case, first half of 14th century, and detail.

base, with the apex pointing upwards. Towards the end of the fourteenth century however, it comes increasingly to be held by the tip, with the base on the upper side, the earliest example being the (flaming) heart in the hands of Caritas on a panel painted by Giovanni del Biondo in circa 1360 (fig.38). From around 1400 onwards, the heart is found more and more frequently as an attribute associated with saints like Augustine, Ansanus, Catherine of Siena, Antony of Padua, and Thomas Aquinas. Some of them have the attribute of a flaming heart, like the earlier Caritas figures. [45]

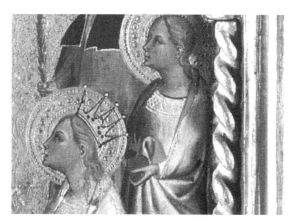

Fig.38. Giovanni del Biondo, *Caritas,* about 1360.

43

THE SCALLOPED HEART

The pine-cone-shaped heart had only a brief life in the arts, its appearance being concentrated in the first half of the fourteenth century. Thereafter, it is only found sporadically. Around 1320, the widely read didactic poem Documenti d'amore by the Florentine jurist Francesco Barberino was circulating. One of the illustrations to that poem features a naked Amor on the back

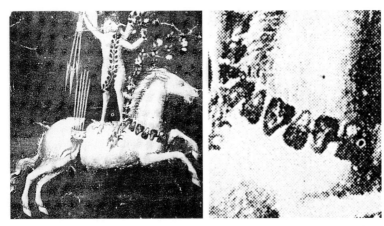

Fig.39. Illustration from Francesco Barberino's *Documenti d'amore*, before 1320, and detail.

of a leaping horse (fig.39). He throws arrows and roses at the bystanders. The hearts are not strung over his shoulder, but around the horse's neck, and they are clearly scalloped. The reproduction of Giotto's Amor (fig.36 on page 42) and the horse from Barberino's book are pictured almost side by side in Panofsky's study on the blind Cupid. Amor's hearts are threaded; they look more like fruit on a tendril than as scalps on a belt, and with one or two of them, there is a small stalk and a very slight dent, as is the case with many fruits. Nevertheless, there is no doubt that here pine-cone-shaped hearts are meant. On the other hand, the hearts around the neck of Barberino's horse remind one in no way of fruit; they lack a stalk and, 'inexplicably', there is clearly a dent in the base.

At the time of the writing of his study in the 1930s, Panofsky had apparently not noticed the intriguing difference between the pine-cone-shaped hearts from Assisi (circa 1323, fig.36 on page 42) and the scalloped hearts in Barberino's book dating from the same period (fig.39). If he had looked more closely at the shape of the heart in Northern Italian art after 1300, he would have noticed the fact that this dip was introduced before or during the making of the coloured pen drawings for Barberino's book, perhaps already before 1320. And in that case, he would probably not simply have suggested a prehistoric origin for the dip in the contour of the heart in his letter of 1961.

Barberino had studied in Florence and Bologna. The miniatures in his book, on which he exerted a strong personal influence, can be classified stylistically as belonging to the school of book illustrators of Bologna, the international centre for anatomical knowledge at the time. Shortly after his book was finished, the scalloped heart also occurs elsewhere in the visual arts, perhaps already in the heart shown in Balduccio's Caritas in figure 33 on page 41. It would seem that the indentation in the left side of this flaming pine-cone-shaped heart is the plastic effect of the pressure of the right child's head. Although unlikely, it is just conceivable that this is an early scalloped heart, the indented base of which would then be concealed under the child's head. Whatever, examples of scalloped hearts are to be found in tapestries dating from the second half of the fourteenth century (fig.40).[46]

The scalloped heart icon is not derived from the hearts on playing cards, because that came about later. According to some scholars, the figures featuring on to-day's playing cards are a development of symbols used during the fifteenth century on Italian cards; here too the heart-icon derived from figures used to represent vases or beakers. According to others, they first made their appearance in France and Germany, but there too the

45

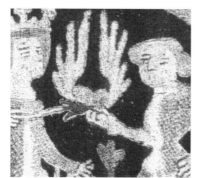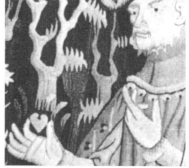

Fig.40. Winged scalloped heart in a German tapestry, about 1400, and a fovea in the heart base on a French tapestry, early 15th century.

'hearts' on the cards were not originally designed with the intention of representing an actual heart. They also arose through a stylisation of other, earlier vignettes, such as vases or pitchers. Only from the end of the fourteenth century was the meaning of a heart projected onto these leaf-shaped vignettes.[47]

Heraldic 'hearts' developed from other forms, equally so, in the main, from leaf motifs. There are medieval shields which we would now call heart-shaped, but which had nothing to do with the heart (fig.41). They may have originated in Italy from the orb regularly

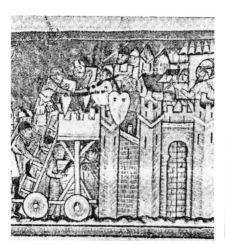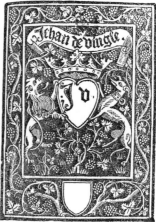

Fig.41. Illustration from *Gran Conquista de Ultramar*, 14th century, and the printer's device of Jehan de Vingle, 1500.

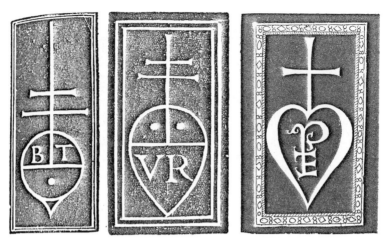

Fig.42. Printers' marks of Baptista de Tortis, 1485, Ugo Rugerius, 1501, and Pierre Levet, 1486.

featured in printers' marks. Devices with variants on this orbiculate form first appeared in the 1480s, such as the one with a dot or pointed base like that of Baptista de Tortis (fig.42), or the shield shape like the one in the device of Ugo Rugerius. Around that time, the heart-icon shape also appeared in printers' devices, perhaps the earliest being that of Pierre Levet.[48]

As the shape of the conical hearts in thirteenth- and fourteenth-century Italian art had been derived from descriptions provided by classical and medieval anatomists, it seems equally logical to look for the source of the dent in contemporary texts and plates in use for anatomical lectures. A source of this kind might well be found in an, as yet undiscovered, text or illustration from an early fourteenth-century anatomist from Bologna, such as Mondeville or Mundinus. But we only find our first scalloped heart in an anatomical work in one of the sixteen plates in the *Anathomia designata per figuras*, of 1345, by their younger contemporary and colleague, the Northern Italian surgeon Guido de Vigevano (fig.43). His description of the heart did not deviate from that of his predecessors (Avicenna, Mondeville and Mundinus). But something had changed in the way its contour is

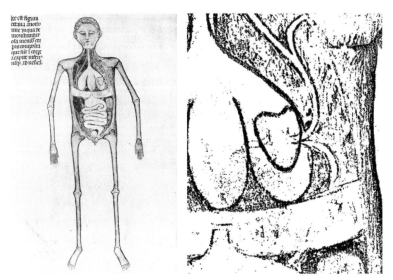

Fig.43. Plate 7 from Guido de Vigevano's *Anothomia designata per figuras*, 1345, and detail of the thoracic cavity.

depicted; here the heart is shown, for the first time in the anatomical literature, with a dent in the base.[49]

One could speculate that anatomists at this time had come to believe that, although a heart is shaped like a pine-cone, it should also show the dent as in a peach. It would then be natural to attribute this transfiguration to the influence of Plutarch's comparison of the heart with a peach. However, none of the medical or other scholarly sources on the heart contains any reference to him. Here and there the classical literature mentions the 'double apex' of a monkey's heart, but the term 'apex' referred to the conical tip of the heart, not to the wide and convex base. Besides, the double apex was not mentioned at all in the medieval treatises.[50]

But then, would it not have been logical simply to depict a two-chambered organ with a dent in its contour? After all, that was the case with the uterus, which classical authors also (mistakenly) took to consist of two compartments. Galen, following Hippocrates, even employed the plural (*uteri*):

You can separate the two uteri from one another and free the one from the other easily (...) It is for this reason that the uterus is named with two names. One of these follows the number which the Grammarians call the 'singular', and the organ is called 'the uterus'. The other follows the number which they call plural, and it is then called 'the uteri'.

We find similar views in Plato and Aristotle and in numerous medical texts down to the middle ages. The fourteenth-century alchemist Gratheus represents the two-chambered uterus (pregnant in this case) with the two-lobed shape that we associate with the icon of the heart, and it is still represented in a scalloped form at the end of the fifteenth century in the *Isagogae breves*

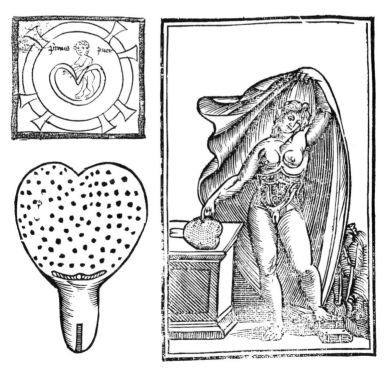

Fig.44. Miniature of a pregnant uterus from Gratheus' didactic poem, 14th century, and woodcuts from Jacopo Berengario's *Isagogae breves*, about 1490.

by Jacopo Berengario (fig.44). The caption to this woodcut runs: 'In the fundus of the uterus there is a certain depression, as you see. This depression distinguishes the right sinus from the left'.[51]

Taking the anology of the uterus which was considered in the middle ages to be composed of two chambers, one could suggest that the heart was also shown with indented base. But this would then prompt the question why it did not occur any earlier than the first decades of the fourteenth century, since by then the heart in its rounded form had made its appearance. Contrary to that of the uterus, that particular shape had been consistently described for a thousand years, namely as a pine-cone with a rounded base. Not a single text on the heart ever mentioned a dent or a 'certain depression'. Albertus Magnus even explicitly wrote that the base of the heart is *indivisum*, undivided. Until the beginning of the fourteenth century, the heart was always represented entirely in accordance with the texts.[52]

Thus, we must look elsewhere for the reason why the pine-cone heart was (relatively) suddenly supplanted by a differently shaped heart. The miniature in Francesco Barberino's book of 1320 certainly depicts scalloped hearts. Was this the first example? We do not know. If it was not, it seems reasonable to assume, therefore, that the changeover must only have been initiated at some point during the preceding years of that century. Since the heart at that time was rarely if ever featured in either the visual arts or literature, the likely explanation must be sought in the field of medicine, and specifically among anatomists, since they had long been the traditional source for the shape given to both the heart and other human organs.

THE THIRD HEART CHAMBER

By the thirteenth century, the university of Bologna had become a centre of medical activities, including the dissection of human cadavers. This 'experimental' interest, however, was the result not so much of an increasing interest in direct observation or a search for new knowledge, as of the need to show and demonstrate what the scholars of antiquity had written. More than ever, the ancient texts were studied in detail, taught and illustrated, and their authority was then still so unassailable that any possible deviation arising from direct observation of the human body was consequently adjusted. It is ironic that, despite the burgeoning interest in anatomy and dissection, we shall see that incorrect assertions about the structure of the heart in two of Aristotle's texts may explain the origin of the dent in its base. Besides the passage cited from the *History of animals* (see page 13), he wrote in *Parts of animals* that, in large mammals, to which man also belongs, the heart has not two but three cavities, and that there is 'an odd one in the middle' between the other two. The exact position of the third chamber, however, could not clearly be identified or visualized on the basis of Aristotle's descriptions.[53]

Galen, an even greater authority than Aristotle in medical matters, explicitly denied the existence of the third chamber. 'What wonder', he wrote, 'that Aristotle, among his many anatomical errors, thinks that the heart in large animals has three cavities'. He considered that what Aristotle had taken to be a third chamber was in fact a cavity (*fovea* in the medieval Latin texts) in the right-hand chamber, in the broad base of the heart. One can understand what led Aristotle to make such a mistake. The anatomy of the heart is complex and confusing, and different cross-sections of the organ can suggest different structures. If, for instance, Aristotle had seen a cross-section such as in figure 45, it is understandable that he would have concluded that there was a third ventricle in the middle of the heart base. Later anatomists, in looking at similar cross-sections of the heart, perhaps saw confirmation of the existence of this 'third ventricle'. It is not surprising, therefore, that Galen's repeated, and correct, criticism of the existence of a third chamber

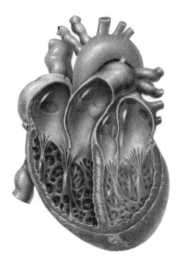

Fig.45. A modern cross-section of the heart, suggesting that three cavities are to be found at the base. The middle one is the exit of the pulmonary artery from the right heart chamber.

failed to call the accuracy of Aristotle's postulation into question until late in the sixteenth century.[54]

About 1000, Avicenna sought to resolve the conflicting classical texts by inserting Aristotle's third ventricle into Galen's heart, thereby disregarding the former's literal text and treating the third chamber as the smallest one, positioning it between the two larger chambers: 'In the heart are three cavities; two large, and a third as it were central in position'. He added that there is a passage between the large right-hand and left-hand chambers. The first translator of Avicenna's *Canon*, Gerard of Cremona, whose work appeared towards the end of the twelfth century, 'improved' on the original by explicitly identifying Galen's fovea with Aristotle's third chamber:

> In it [the heart] are three ventricles; two are large, and the third as it were between, which Galen called the fovea or non-ventricular meatus, so that there may be a receptaculum for the thick and strong nourishment, like to the substance of the

heart, with which it is nourished, and also a storehouse for the pneuma (spiritus) generated in it from the subtil blood. And between the two are channels or meatuses.[55]

One of the earliest medieval books on the subject, is *De motu cordis,* by Alfredus Anglicus around 1210:

The heart is divided into three chambers (...) and rests on the base, closed off by a small chamber (...). Aristotle refers to this hollow opening *(meatus)* as the middle chamber, primarily because it has in its centre a large and deep cavity *(profundam habeat concavitum).*

Pointing to Galen, Anglicus observed that the classical physicians had not reached a consensus on the subject, but he continued further with Aristotle's text.

Similar passages are to be found in another work of the same period, in which the anatomical doctrine of Aristotle is even more prominently represented, viz. the *Anatomia vivorum* (circa 1225), which is thought to have been written by a Salernitan doctor called Ricardus. He also mentioned Galen's dissenting opinion about the third chamber, here followed by the teaching of Avicenna. But the writer made no attempt to address or clarify the differing accounts, nor does he appear to understand what is meant by an opening, called fovea:

Between these chambers is a central opening called fovea by the authors, situated in the base of the heart, in which the blood is mixed with air, making vital spirits which the heart forces through all the organs of the body.[56]

His contemporary, Albertus Magnus, on the other hand, did point out the contradiction between the Aristotelian and Galenic texts, but did not suggest a solution either:

> (...) there are three chambers in the wide section of the heart. Aristotle calls the chamber in the centre the middle chamber, in which, as he states, the process of nourishment is completed. Galen, however, calls the middle one a cavity instead of a chamber (*fovea non ventriculus*).

A similar description is to be found in the 'encyclopedia' by Bartholomaeus Anglicus, written about 1260.[57]

Mondeville also placed the third chamber 'in between the two chambers, in a partition, in the middle of which is a cavity called 'third chamber' by some'. In his sketch of the heart, the third chamber is therefore drawn in the middle, but in this case it is situated not at the base but at the tip of the heart (fig.46). It is not clear why he

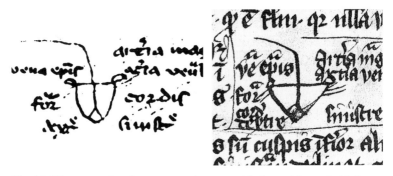

Fig.46. Diagrams of a pine-cone and a pyramid-shaped heart (with heart ears) from 14th-century manuscripts of Henri de Mondeville's *Anatomie*.

thought that the third chamber was situated there. The anatomical sources which considered its location in more detail all state that the third chamber is situated on the upper side of the heart, in the middle of the wide base. The small area at the tip of Mondeville's heart could at first sight be taken to be an illustration of the Hippocratic 'solid apex, being, as it were, stitched onto the outside', but Mondeville clearly intended to depict the third ventricle there, as can be seen from his own French translation of the original Latin text:

> The heart has two ventricles, i.e. two chambers (...). In between those two concavities is a partition, and in the middle of this partition at the lower side is a concavity that some call the third ventricle.

It is conceivable that this misunderstanding about the localization of the third ventricle in the heart point dates back to an earlier text, such as, for example, that of Alfredus Anglicus (see quotation on page 53), who wrote that the heart 'rests on the base, closed off by a small chamber'. It is easy to understand the confusion about what constituted the top and the base of the heart. In the classical literature, the broad upper section of the pine-cone-shaped heart was referred to as the base of the heart. Taking the word literally, some medieval scribes assumed that the base lay at the lower section of the heart and thus, understandably but incorrectly, they identified the base with the point underneath. The same confusion existed in Avicenna's work, when he wrote that 'the base of the right chamber descends much lower'.[58]

Johannes Mesue even thought that the three chambers of the heart are not arranged horizontally side by side, but are vertically stacked:

> The [heart] has three pouches as some purses do; air is received into the uppermost, blood into the lower pouch, and the one in between (called *fovea*) is where the mixing of air and blood and the quickening of the spirits takes place.[59]

Neither Mondeville's low positioning of the third chamber at the tip of the heart nor Mesue's placement in the middle of the vertical axis convinced their colleagues.

Confusion persisted, however, as can also be seen from the work of their contemporary Mundinus. He described the operation of the middle chamber 'miraculous because it consists not of one large but of many small concavities, which are broader in the right-hand chamber than in the left-hand one'. In the same book, he wrote that the heart consists of three chambers, the third being situated between the two large chambers, lying 'in the thickness of the *septum*', the vertical partition separating the two large chambers. We also find Galenus' phrasing: 'duos ventriculos, dextrum et sinistrum, et in medio foveam' (the latter being translated in Middle English as 'it has in the middle a ditch or pit') in the surgical manual produced by Guy de Chauliac.[60]

The medieval anatomists had to make do with faulty translations or texts copied from generation to generation, often by scribes who had no understanding of their contents. The descriptions of the third chamber were inconsistent and for centuries had a confusing influence on the topography of the heart. This perplexity is hardly surprising, however, since the third chamber does not exist. At most, some semblance of harmonisation with the classical texts was achieved.

Aristotle had localized the third chamber inside the heart, as did Galen his fovea. But, as we have seen, its form and placement were no longer clear in the medieval summaries of their works: in the middle of the heart, in all probability at the base thereof, there is an opening called a hollow or ditch, which is not a chamber but rather an open chamber, a vault, a concavity or a pit.[61]

An anatomist or artist soon after 1300 who attempted to reconcile these descriptions in a diagram would have had an impossible task, even if he had had the complete classical anatomical sources at his disposal. The available contemporary texts were short, superficial and often self-contradictory. None of these descriptions would have enabled the reader to be certain exactly where the concavity was located, nor if what was meant was inside the heart or whether it was a dent in the external side. Even if there had been any interest at all in the factual reality, dissection would not have provided any justification for either interpretation. That use of the word 'concavity' could be taken to indicate an indentation in an organ is evident from Chauliac's description of the gall-bladder, which lies in an external niche of the liver: 'the gall-bladder is a purse (...) set in the concavity of the liver'.62

It is obvious that an anatomist who wished to draw a heart could represent the fovea as a dip in the outside wall of its base, like, for example, the one in the heart in the second picture of figure 40 on page 46. But even if it was the intention to depict not the fovea but the smaller third ventricle between the two larger ones in the broad base of the pine-cone-shaped heart, it would have only been natural to introduce a dip or indentation into the rounded upper line of its contour.

The triangular dip in the middle of the base of the isolated eleventh-century Cambridge heart sketch (fig.15 on page 26) is the oldest known illustration of the fovea or the third chamber. It is situated exactly where it ought to be, according to the text of the *Anatomia vivorum* and other medical sources. Here the presence of the third chamber creates a triangular indentation in the cross-section of the base of the heart. There is no reason for assuming, however, that this astrological sketch could have had any effect on the external dent which occurred more than two centuries later in Vigevano's 'anatomical' heart.

Anatomists used to illustrate their lessons with anatomical sketches (like those in figures 18, 21, 22 on pages 29, 31, 32), but no illustration of the heart is to be found in any of the numerous medieval copies and editions of Mundinus' famous textbook of anatomy. The first illustration of it is to be found in a printed version of Mundinus' *Anathomia* published by Johannes Adelphus in 1513 (fig.47). In this figure, the third chamber is situated

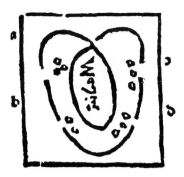

Fig.47. Cross-section of the heart from the printed edition of Mundinus' anatomy book by Adelphus, 1513.

in the middle between the two large chambers, in the wide part of the heart, the place where it was supposed to lie according to the majority of the anatomical sources. This sketch also indicates a 'passage' between the right-hand and left-hand chambers, as described by Aristotle in a rather obscure text, and Avicenna echoed this: 'the heart has a receptacle [the right ventricle] for the nutriment, a place where the pneuma is formed [the left ventricle] and thirdly, a canal between the two'.[63]

Adelphus used this diagram to explain how the 'circulation of the blood' operates. For this purpose, he used the diagram indicating the openings, the heart valves and the *ostia*. The illustration may be a copy of an older sketch, used as a teaching aid perhaps by Mundinus himself, who, according to Adelphus, was being worshipped, even as late as the sixteenth century, as a veritable deity. The woodcutter faithfully engraved the original sketch in the wood-block, but he did not grasp its significance, because he literally copied the word *Medium*, which referred to the third ventricle, so that the original pen drawing from the manuscript appeared as a mirror image in the printed book. Adelphus had obviously not understood the original either, or perhaps he was not disturbed by the mistake, since there is no reference to the diagram in his accompanying text. Nor did he mention the third ventricle as described in Mundinus' original text, but he did follow it in referring

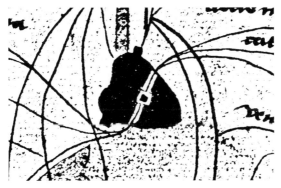

Fig.48. First scalloped heart, in a five-picture series, late 14th century. See also figure 22.

to the openings. He further described only the function of the arteries and veins that originate in the heart, although they do not appear in the sketch.

Early printed anatomical works that were based on medieval manuscripts contain woodcuts of scalloped hearts, no doubt taken from illustrations in those earlier manuscripts. The first scalloped heart in one of the traditional five-picture series is to be found towards the end of the fourteenth century (fig.48). An illustration from the printed *Anthropologium* by the Leipzig physician Magnus Hundt also shows a scalloped Vigevano heart contour (fig.49), and the cross-section of the heart from the *Compendium* of Johannes Peyligk illustrates how the dip is connected with the third chamber, i.e. in the same way as in the Adelphus edition of Mundinus' *Anathomia* (fig.47). Compared with these illustrations of the heart, done by anatomists who slavishly accepted the anatomical texts of their predecessors, Leonardo's sketch, apparently based on direct observation, looks positively modern.[64]

The origin of the dip in the contour of the base of the heart must have been facilitated by the drawing of the vertical *sulcus longitudinalis* (or *sulcus interventricularis*) in anatomical sketches. This is a vertical furrow on the outside of the heart that corresponds to the internal

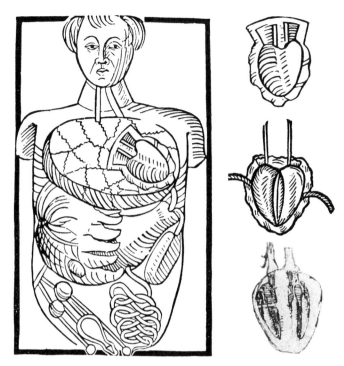

Fig.49. Heart sketches from Magnus Hundt's *Anthropologium*, 1501, from the 1499 edition of Johannes Peyligk's *Compendium*, and from Leonardo da Vinci (about 1500).

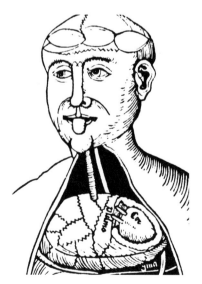

Fig.50. Pine-cone heart from Johannes Peyligk's *Compendium*, 1516.

attachment of the septum, the partition between the two chambers. It can be seen in Hundt's heart and in the Vesalian hearts (figs.49 and 85 on page 101).[65]

The question that remains is what the first dip in the first scalloped heart looked like: was it a round, concave indentation, a fovea, or was it an acute fold or an obtuse angle? The indentations in the first known artistic representations of the heart in Barberino's treatise (fig.38) are both concave and angular, while that in the first known anatomical representation, in Vigevano's book, was concave. If the original sketch, from which the woodcut in the Adelphus edition of Mundinus' anatomy book (fig.47 on page 58) was derived, dates from shortly after 1300, an angular indentation would have been the first of the two.

A possible explanation for the primacy of the sharp dent may be that the third ventricle, which older sources placed on the upper side of the base of the heart – as can be seen in the Cambridge heart (fig.15 on page 26) – was situated by later anatomists at a lower level of the central line, midway between the base and the apex, as in the Pisa heart (fig.18 on page 29). This could have prompted them to repeat the dip in the base as a more acute, angular incision. In that case, the concave dip would have been a somewhat later stylisation of it.

An early French example of a heart icon with a more angular dip, or even a fold, in the base can be seen on a seal showing a heart with an 'arterial tree' and a cross (fig.51). The arterial tree is a stylised representation of a metaphor of Galen, who wrote that 'from the heart springs out an artery in the same manner as does the trunk of a tree from the earth' and just like 'the trunk of the tree divides into branches'. In the second half of the fourteenth century, the heart surmounted by a cross, which 'grew out' of the arterial tree, came to represent the Sacred heart, while the previous image of the tree which is growing from the base of the heart, remained.[66]

61

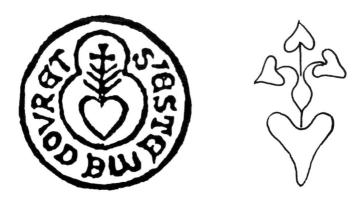

Fig.51. Heart with angular indentation in the base and convex sides in the seal of Esteme Couret, late 14th century, and a heart with arterial tree in a watermark, 16th century.

WATERMARK HEARTS, THE CLOVEN HEART

Deeply scalloped figures, shaped like the heart icon, already appeared in the watermarks of Italian paper manufacturers in the first half of the fourteenth century. The oldest known example is in a document dating from 1326 found in Le Puy in the south of France (fig.52). It consists of an elongated triangle with curved corners, intersected in the middle by two dotted lines, and with a deep indentation between the two upper corners. The same is true of a watermark in the paper of a document

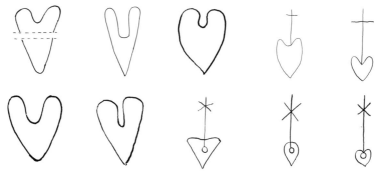

Fig.52. The heart icon as a watermark dated, from left to right, 1326, 1330, 1396, 1404, 1417, 1442, 1468, 1470, 1495, and 1564.

from 1330 in Grenoble; this figure has a very tapered point below and a very wide and deep indentation on the upper side. It is generally assumed that these early contours were intended to represent not a heart but a leaf.[67]

Increasingly, in the course of the fourteenth century, however, these figures came to assume the less deeply scalloped form, and by the end of the century, hundreds of these 'leaf-shaped' watermarks in Italian and French paper came more and more to resemble our modern heart icon. Some of them included an arrow, others a crown (fig.53). Although watermarks with leaf ornaments (spade leaves or clover leaves) continued to

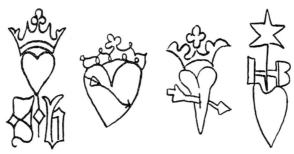

Fig.53. Crowned hearts in watermarks, 16th century.

be used down to the present, it seems more natural, if one surveys the continuous development of these figures, to suppose that the earliest watermarks in the primitive form of the heart icon were already intended to show a heart with a fovea. The crude manner in which watermarks were drawn serves to explain the sometimes extreme shape of these hearts. The horizontal lines in one of the figures could indicate the coronary arteries, which entwine the heart like a garland at about this level. Its source can also be found in a Galenic text: 'There are two arteries coursing around in a circle through the body of the heart'. The image of the crown of the heart was also used by Galen: 'the circular base of the pericardium [i.e. the membranous sac which encloses the heart] surrounds the base of the heart like a crown'.[68]

Two of the watermarks illustrated in figure 52 display a heart with an unusually deep indentation. In a manuscript dating from the first half of the fifteenth century, there is a drawing of *Pietas* (Compassion) holding a very large split heart (*cor scissum in duas partes*) in his hand (fig.54). It shows

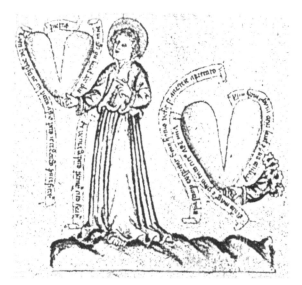

Fig.54. *Pietas*, first half of the 15th century.

that God has 'a cloven heart because of his love for us. Thus, man must also have a cloven heart, i.e. Compassion. He must be ready to meet the needs of his neighbours, particularly the poor and the infirm.' This heart seems to have been cleaved in two from above. We encounter this image in a courtly love poem by the thirteenth-century Italian poet, Guido Guinizelli, which speaks of Amor's arrow splitting the heart of the lover in two:

> For he shot an arrow through my heart's centre
> That cuts one part from the other and divides the
> whole.

Such a cleft heart appeared in 1575 above a money-chest in an emblem of Bernardus Furmerius (fig.55). Coins fall through the split in the heart instead of into the chest. The meaning is that true richness must fill hearts and not chests. The same picture can be found on a German altarpiece by Hans Fries dating from 1506. Meanwhile the translator of Furmerius' book of emblems, Dirck Coornhert, had also used it in two prints, in which the Penitent literally tears the heart open and in so doing manifests his remorse and sadness.[69]

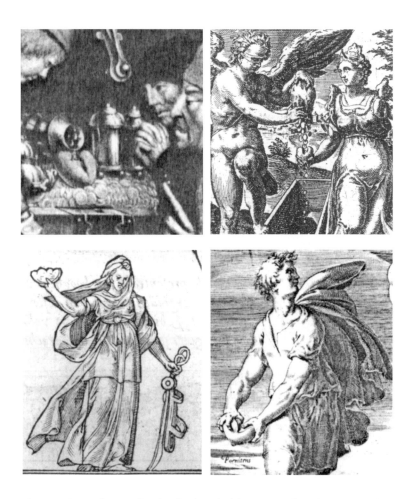

Fig.55. Cloven heart of a dead miser in his money-chest by Hans Fries, 1506, cloven heart above a money-chest in an emblem by Bernardus Furmerius, 1575, *Reason's* unfolded heart by Jean Houwaert, 1579, and Dirck Coornhert, *Poenitens*, about 1580.

The cloven heart of the fifteenth-century Pietas is not necessarily an extreme shape of the scalloped heart icon; it is a quite separate representation. Its provenance is unclear. It may have originated, directly or indirectly, from one or two passages in the Bible, particularly in the Book of Psalms, where a broken heart is associated with *Pietas*: compassion, mercy, kindness, tenderness and righteousness. Representations of cloven hearts also occurred later, by cleaving a scalloped heart, as is clear from the upper edge of the opened heart of Reason in figure 55. The symbolic meaning of the cloven heart, at least in the sixteenth century, is no longer unambiguous, as may appear from the symbol of openheartedness in the hand of this allegorical figure.[70]

The trachea heart

After about 1400, the dent in the heart base was gratefully used by illustrators who knew it was in there that the entrance to the hollow heart was situated. This is hardly surprising, as Aristotle wrote that the windpipe *(trachea)*, leads not only to the lungs, but also to the heart. Galen describes no fewer than three large vessels that connect the base of the heart with the lung, but the widest and most striking of these he calls the 'rough artery', i.e. the trachea, the wall of which is reinforced with cartilage rings. It branches 'into all the parts of the lung, being distributed along with the vessels from the heart into all the lobes'. The heart is thus supplied with air because it is transported from the small branches of the trachea into the small branches of the blood vessels (i.e. of the 'smooth artery'). This air is turned into *pneuma* in the heart. Although this description of the oxydization of the blood is roughly accurate, Galen's account of the exact anatomical link between the trachea and the heart is so unclear (not to say incorrect) that it could have given rise to the mistaken belief that the former is linked directly to the latter.[71]

According to Galen and to authors in the middle ages, the lungs do not have a direct respiratory function; they play a secondary role compared with the bronchial tubes. As we have seen with respect to the hazelnut heart, the lung tissue also played a subordinate role compared to the heart. It was merely considered as a 'spongy substance like padding to fill up the empty spaces between all the vessels and be a support and safeguard for the weakness at that point (...). As long as [the trachea] has not stopped dividing, the flesh of the lung must grow about it'. The lung had yet another function, and that was to act as a kind of gland that was made to concoct the outer air to acquire a 'quality proper to the innate pneuma'. But it is the windpipe and its branches which are 'connected with the heart' to supply it with air and to serve as an 'exhaust pipe' for the evacuation of its waste matter.[72]

In a number of medieval anatomical prints, it is mainly (and incorrectly) the trachea, as the thickest of the heart 'vessels', which has been retained. Up to the late fifteenth century, it is represented as attached to the heart like a stalk (Albertus Magnus called it a stick) to a spade leaf. The lungs themselves are absent altogether. We have seen such trachea hearts, without the lungs, in some of the ancient Egyptian representations of the heart (fig.7 on page 12), and in hearts in medieval five-picture Circulation men. A nice example of a trachea heart in the arts is the miser's heart in a relief by Donatello (1447), illustrating a passage from Luke (12:34): 'For where your treasure is, there will be your heart also'. The heart found in the money-chest of the dead miser was here represented with a trachea heart instead of a simple conical one (fig.56). Even after Vesalius, these incorrect anatomical drawings did not disappear. In Hans von Gersdorff's mid-sixteenth-century surgery book, there is a diagram in which the trachea is represented as opening directly into the heart. A late example is found in an eighteenth- century Chinese medical text.[73]

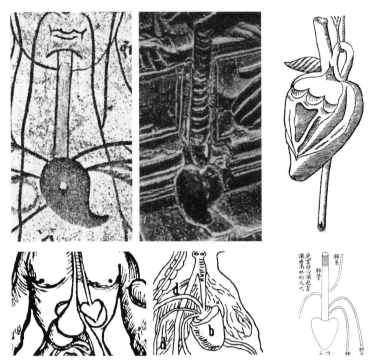

Fig.56. Trachea hearts without lungs. Top row: from a Circulation man in the Caius five-picture series, early 13th century, from the money-chest of Donatello's *Miracle of the heart of the miser*, 1447, and from the surgery book by Hans von Gersdorff, 1556. Lower row: from a Wound man, about 1485, from a Chinese anatomical atlas, 16th century, and from the 18th-century Chinese *Imperial encyclopedia*.

While the origin of the trachea heart dates back to classical anatomical texts, the more extensive trachea-lung-heart specimens, sometimes including the abdominal organs, as seen in figure 11, originate in ancient religious rites. The organs of sacrificial animals had to be 'read' and the messages from the gods had to be interpreted from them. A good example is the scene on an Etruscan bronze mirror from the fifth century BC (fig.57) on which a haruspex is inspecting a liver, while a trachea-lung-heart preparation lies on the table in front of him. The oval outline in front of the lung lobe is the heart. It might well be argued that the Etruscan trachea hearts have their ultimate origin in those created by the Ancient Egyptians; two examples of the latter feature in figure 7 on page 12 .[74]

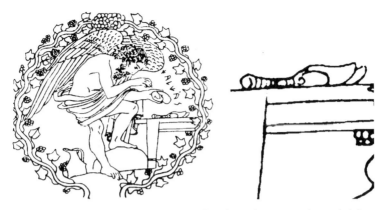

Fig.57. Etruscan bronze mirror. A trachea-lung-heart specimen is lying on the table.

The heart is intimately connected with the lung by three pairs of large blood vessels, originating in the heart base and branching out like a tree into the entire lung tissue. From above, the bronchial tubes also branch out downwards from the trachea into the lung. This makes it relatively easy during the slaughtering of animals, or in human dissection, to remove the heart and lungs together from the thorax by cutting the windpipe in the throat and detaching the lungs and the heart in one piece from the surrounding tissues. It was, therefore, logical to remove these organs from the thoracic cavity in their entirety. That this also occurred is clear from the post mortem conducted on Pope Alexander v, following his sudden death in Bologna on 4 May 1410. The surgeon, Pietro d'Argellata, wrote: 'I now passed to the spiritual members [i.e. the thorax] and removed lung and heart and all their ligaments.' The trachea can then be gripped like a stalk to which both the lungs and heart are attached below like a piece of meat. A trachea-heart-lung specimen can also be found in the books of the anatomists who carried out dissections, e.g. in Vesalius' *Fabrica* and Casserio's *De vocis* (fig.58).[75]

The magical trachea-lung-heart specimen of the Etruscan haruspex in later centuries also acquired the characteristics of an ex-voto or symbol of the heart proper.

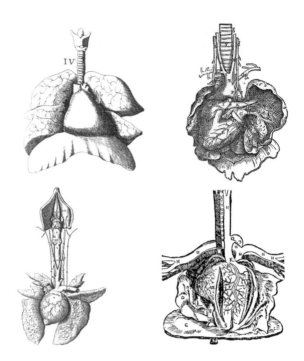

Fig.58. Trachea-lung-heart specimens from the anatomy books of Dryander, 1540, Vesalius, 1543 (seen from behind), Eustachius, ca. 1552, and Casserio, 1601, three of which have part of the diaphragm attached.

Such a (trachea, lung and heart) specimen of the organs of the thorax appears next to the isolated heart, as an attribute of Ansanus, one of the patron saints of Siena (fig.59). It seems as though the heart and the combination of trachea, heart and lung (occasionally with liver and stomach) were sometimes considered symbolic equivalents and were interchangeable as late as the sixteenth century.[76]

THE PITCHER HEART

The association of the heart with a pitcher had already been made in Ancient Egypt (see fig. 7 on page 12). The pitcher-shaped heart, with a neck protruding from the (now dented) upper contour, made its appearance at the beginning of the fifteenth century. This development is no doubt the result of the fact that the heart is hollow, a

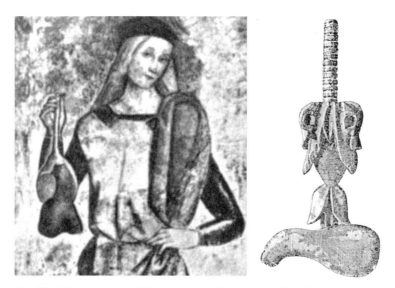

Fig.59. Saint Ansanus holding a trachea-lung-heart-liver (or stomach) ex-voto, 15th century. The heart is the grey egg-shaped organ at the left. Right: one of the contemporary polyvisceral ex-votos, which appear in churches in Bavaria and the Tyrol region.

vessel to which a piece of the trachea, or one of the large blood-vessels which emerge from its base, had remained attached. In addition, as in the case of the hearts on playing cards, the shape of the ornamental calyx of a flower and similarly-shaped pottery, like the flaming vase in a twelfth-century mosaic in the San Clemente basilica in Rome (fig.60), may have had an influence too. Such

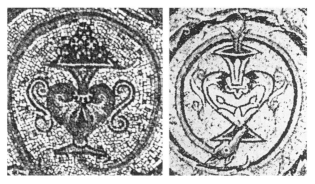

Fig.60. Mosaic of the Triumph of the cross, in the apse of the upper basilica of San Clemente, Rome, first half of the 12th century.

associations of similar visual forms, and their mutual impact on the human mind, must have induced Panofsky to postulate a *Gestalt*-psychological process for the way in which the 'schematization' into what we now call the heart-shaped form came about. As a result of all these influences, a new iconographical heart shape emerged: a pitcher with a neck, often with a lip.[77]

The image of the heart as a hollow or abode in which the loved one resides regularly features in courtly poetry from the twelfth century onwards. An explicit early literary source for the heart-pitcher metaphor appeared about 1200 in a poem by Hartmann von Aue, in which the man's love sickness is treated by pouring a herbal mixture into the heart:

> he should pour it into a jar:
> that is a heart without hate.

These lines were copied and quoted down to the sixteenth century.[78]

Through the contamination of the images of heart and vessel it is not always clear where the precise dividing

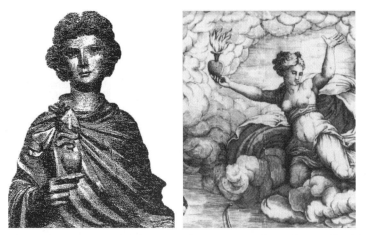

Fig.61. Saint Ansanus with heart pitcher, 1400, and Baccio Bandinelli's *Venus*, 1545.

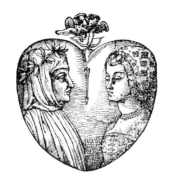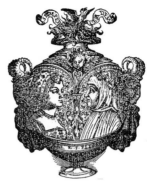

Fig.62. Vignette on the title-pages of Petrarch's *Sonetti*, 1544 and 1550.

line can be drawn between a heart-shaped vessel and a pitcher-shaped heart. We have a heart-shaped pitcher around 1400 in the hand of Saint Ansanus (fig.61). In the course of the fifteenth century, he was partly replaced by Saint Catherine, who, like him, as a patron saint of the city, was increasingly pictured with a heart as an attribute. Although there are a number of examples of Ansanus as baptist with a water vessel, it is conceivable that the heart pitcher in figure 61 really represents a heart. We find such a (flaming) heart vessel held by Venus in an engraving by Baccio Bandinelli. Here, as with the Ratisbon Caritas in figure 26 on page 36, the pitcher and the heart appear to be interchangeable. Such a pitcher heart appears later in the hands of Saint Catherine of Siena and of Saint Augustine. The close association of

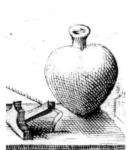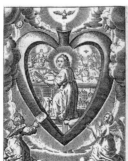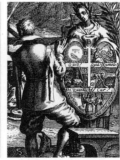

Fig.63. *Coeur trompeur* from Velde's *Openhertighe herten*, about 1620, hearts from Antoine Suquet's *Den wegh des eewich levens*, 1620, and Etienne Luzuic's *Cor Deo devotum*, 1628.

heart and vase can also be seen, for example, in their mutual interchangeability in the printer's mark in two editions of the poems of Petrarch (fig.62).[79]

Later, especially after 1600, this heart shape became popular when Anton Wierix made a series of prints of a large hollow heart in which the Child Jesus featured as *Amor divinus* (fig.63). Some of these hearts are so big that they look like a cave whose opening rises up into the air like a chimney from the dip in the base, so that their form becomes virtually identical to that of the ancient vase ornaments (fig.60). The influence of pitcher shapes on the contour of the heart was one of the factors leading to the emergence in the 1620s of the emblem books with large pitcher-shaped hearts as those of Benedictus van Haeften, Etienne Luzuic and their many successors.[80]

THE TAPERED HEART ICON

At first, the lower side of the heart icon was portrayed as round as a peach, like the enormous heart in the hands of 'Ame devote' and in other miniatures by the Master of King Rene of Anjou in *Le mortifiement de vaine plaisance* from the middle of the fifteenth century (fig.35 on page 41). This heart is as unrealistically large as the one by

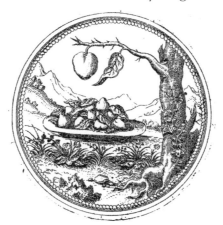

Fig.64. Joachim Camerarius, *Idem ambo*, 1590.

Taddeo Gaddi in the Baroncelli chapel (fig.32 on page 40), where the master may have seen it. Similar peach-shaped hearts, though somewhat smaller, are also to be found in the hand of Amor in the *Livre du cuer d'amours espris* by the same master.[81]

It is not until the sixteenth century, however, that we again find an explicit reference to the Egyptian peach heart in Andrea Alciati's *Emblematum liber* (1531) and in an emblem by the German humanist Joachim Camerarius (fig.64), with the text harking back to Plutarch: *Persea fert cordis fructus, folia aemula linguae, O vtinam in cunctis haec bene juncta forent* ('The peach tree bears fruits that can vie with the heart, leaves that can vie with the tongue. Would that these two were in harmony in all things').[82]

The scalloped heart icon originally had two convex sides. This more or less cone- or peach-shaped contour with a round tip has been current since the fourteenth century, as attributes in the hands of Saint Augustine and of the Northern Italian saints (fig.65). Later, we find an example in the book of emblems by Roemer Visscher from 1614 and contemporaries, like Dirck Coornhert or Hendrick Goltzius. This is also the shape that Erwin

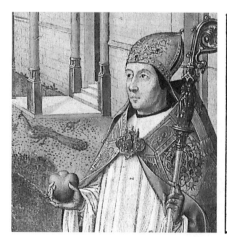 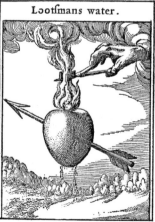

Fig.65. Convex-shaped hearts, in the hand of Saint Augustine, with lip-shaped neck, about 1500, and in an emblem by Roemer Visscher, 1614.

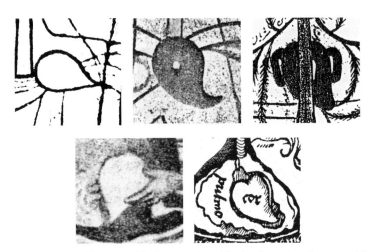

Fig.66. Hearts with a one-sided concavity with the tip pointed to one side, from left to right:12th century Pruefening five-picture heart, early 13th century Caius five-picture heart, late 14th century Persian five-picture heart, late 14th century post mortem heart, and the heart from *Margarita philosophica*, about 1500. See also the Donatello heart in figure 56 on pag 68.

Panofsky drew in his 1961 letter (fig.2 on page 8). Of all heart icon shapes, this convex shape was for centuries the one most usually found, but the icon with concave sides has gradually become more common than the plump form and has perhaps nowadays become the dominant one.[83]

The origin of the concave sides of the heart icon is of later date than the dent in its basis, but a concave contour that is confined to the left-hand side alone of the cone-shaped heart, i.e. a comma-shaped heart contour, already appeared much earlier in the five-picture series (fig.66). This was the consequence of the fact that Galen and his followers stated that the tip of the heart points to the left:

(the heart) lies rather towards the left, since its tip, unlike its base, does not lie precisely midway between the right and the left of the thorax. It is not streched from head to tip precisely in the median line, but it bends slightly, as I have mentioned, towards the left.

76

Sometimes the artist drew this by making the whole pine-cone slant towards the lower left or even horizontal. But the tip of the vertically drawn cone was also often given a push to the left at the bottom; this ensured compliance with the texts of the classical authorities, but even more closely with the text of Mondeville:

> Its tapered side, that is, the point below, bends a little to the left, as the philosopher said in the first book of the *History of animals*, and at the end of the sixth chapter.[84]

An indication of this concavity on the left is already visible in the Pruefening heart (fig.17 on page 28), but it is far more extreme in the heart of the 'circulation man' from the Caius five-picture series (fig.21 on page 31) and in late fourteenth-century five-picture hearts. Another striking example of a heart of this shape is Donatello's trachea heart (fig.56 on page 68). It is also noteworthy how much these hearts with the tip pointing to one side resemble the leaf-shaped ornaments in classical texts and late sixteenth-century books (fig.67).[85]

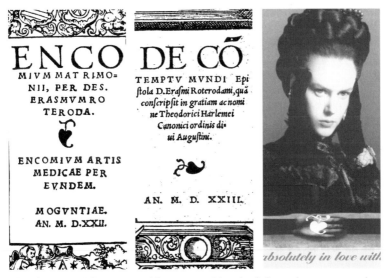

Fig.67. Two 16th-century title pages with a leaf-shaped ornamentation (*hedera*), and the same ornamentation on a modern postcard.

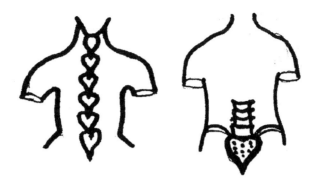

Fig.68. Leaf-shaped vertebrae and sacrum, 14th century.

The scalloped heart icon with symmetrical concave sides and tapering to a sharp point, like the one on contemporary playing cards, became popular in the course of the sixteenth century, and was probably due to the influence of the concave sides of the ornamental ivy leaf, an image, which, for centuries, has exerted its effect on the contour of the pine-cone heart. The classical leaf ornament had an enormous impact on design and decoration in general. In the later middle ages too, leaf contours still affected the shape of representations of other organs besides the heart. For instance, in some primitive anatomical sketches, the bladder, the vertebrae or the sacrum, in the absence of precise knowledge of their correct form, had the contour of a double concave ivy leaf (fig.68), and today we still find ivy leaves used decoratively in modern designs.[86]

That confusion between the leaf shape and the heart icon still occurs can be seen from a recent postcard on which love is symbolised by a leaf ornament (*hedera*) that was used by the early printers, comma-shaped and copied from, or inspired by, similar ornaments in Roman inscriptions. But the designer of the recent postcard mistook it for a stylised representation of the heart (fig.67).

A heart icon with straight sides is a relatively recent manifestation. Contemporary examples are those

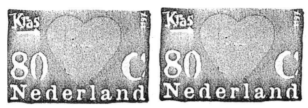

Fig.69. Heart with an angular dip in the base, right sides and a convex point on a Dutch postage stamp, 1997.

featured on a postage stamp issued by the Dutch PTT in 1997 (fig.69) and the logo of a garden exhibition dating from the same year (fig.70). In the latter, the leaf and the heart are represented by the same icon, the leaf and stalk are coloured green, and the 'heart' is red. It conjoins the ancient ornamental spade leaf and the modern heart icon to proclaim the message: 'We love plants'.[87]

The pointed apex of the icon has prevailed over the more rounded lower side of the cone or peach. It is the obvious result of making the sides concave. Apart from that, the learned texts provided a sound basis for furnishing the lower side of a heart sketch with a pointed tip. Aristotle explicitly wrote that 'the apex of the heart

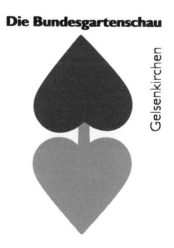

Fig.70. Logo of the Bundesgartenschau 1997, Gelsenkirchen, Germany. The heart-leaves have an angular dip in the base, right sides and a pointed apex. The upper leaf was red, the lower green.

is sharp', Mesue called the lower side a sharp point (*est acutum punctale*), and Chauliac referred to it as the sharpness of the heart'.[88]

To summarize the hypothesis of the origin of the dip in the base of the heart, the conclusion must be that it is the indirect result of a text by Aristotle describing a third chamber of the heart, and of the commentaries on the Latin translation of the passage by Galen, referring to a fovea in the middle of the base. The descriptions provided by the classical authorities were either incorrect, conflicting or unclear. The medieval translators and anatomists were uninterested or confused, which is obvious from their superficial and inconsistent versions of the original texts. Galen's extensive and detailed descriptions were often reduced to a few short statements. It was clearly impossible to represent all the elements in a diagram on the basis of these accounts. Nevertheless, late medieval anatomists and artists introduced a detailed 'refinement' into the classical contour of the heart: a dent appeared in the middle of the rounded base at the spot where the smaller third chamber was supposed to be located.

The dent first appeared in Northern Italy, where classical and translated texts were being intensively studied and taught, in Bologna in particular, from the beginning of the fourteenth century. It does not occur in the thirteenth century. It must have originated after 1304, the year in which Mondeville was still using the pyramidal diagram for his anatomy lectures in Montpellier (fig.46 on page 54).

It is first seen in the visual arts in the miniatures in Barberino's book (fig.39), drawn in Bologna before 1320. It may, however, have occurred before or around 1316, the year in which Mundinus' anatomy book was written. An illustration from this book (or from his courses) may have been the original of the woodcut which later appeared in the printed edition by Adelphus (fig.47 on page 58). The earliest extant illustration of a scalloped heart in an anatomical work is contained in de Vigevano's book of 1347 (fig.43 on page 48). It appeared more frequently as the century progressed, but it did not really come into its own until the early years of the 15th century. The Graeco-Arabic conical heart began to disappear by the second half of the fourteenth century. But the hearts in the old, primitive, 'non-academic' five-picture series continued to be shown in their conical shape, almost without exception, up to the sixteenth century. In 1499, the *Compendium* of Peyligk contains a pine-cone-shaped heart (fig.50) next to a scalloped heart (fig.49 on page 60).[89]

As in anatomy, the pine-cone heart did not disappear from the arts overnight. Around 1425, Fra Angelico was still painting one as an attribute in the hand of a Dominican. Saint Antony of Padua holds a similar heart in his hand in a painting by Fiorenzo di Lorenzo, which dates from circa 1450, as does Saint Catherine of Siena in a sculpture by an unknown master from around 1500. The conical shape was still being encountered in Tibetan temple decorations dating from about 1800.[90]

The 'scallop correction' to the classical conical heart contour was an anatomical heresy that persisted for more than two hundred years. The increasing impact of direct anatomical observation dispelled the belief in the

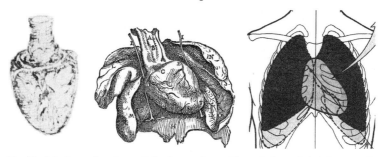

Fig.71. Modern sketches of the heart from (from left to right) Leonardo da Vinci, about 1500, Vesalius, 1543, and *Gray's anatomy*, 1995. (The two vessels protruding up from the base of Vesalius' heart remind one of those in figure 49 on page 60).

existence of the third ventricle and with it, the need for the scalloped contour in anatomical illustrations which did not correspond to reality. Although a real heart can display a variety of forms, depending upon how it is removed from the body and on the angle from which it is viewed, the most appropriate shape to represent its contour remains that of the pine-cone. The anatomical drawings of real hearts made from direct observation by Leonardo, Vesalius and by modern artists thus show the old rounded form (fig.71).[91]

The increase in anatomical knowledge after 1500 did not, however, create a consequential need to dispense with the indentation in what had become the accepted (i.e. both popular and artistic) image of the heart. Clearly, the scalloped heart had become entrenched in the visual arts and it had come to lead a life of its own as a generally recognized symbol, an icon. It was obviously unnecessary (and probably impossible) to amend its shape to conform to its true contour.

Seen from an iconographic perspective, the most striking feature in the story of the shape of the heart is that its textual description has not fundamentally changed in the course of 2500 years, while its visual portrayal has undergone a complex evolution. Although

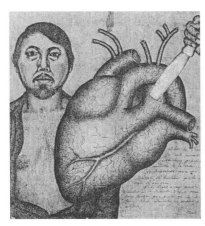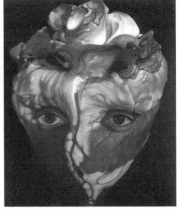

Fig. 72. Nahum Zenil, *Ex-voto*, 1987, and Alain Miller, *Eye love eye*, 1997.

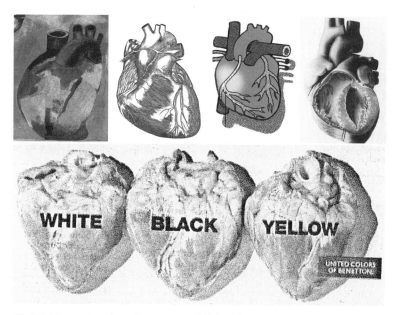

Fig.73. Hearts in advertisements published between 1995 and 1997.

it continued to feature in anatomical works, the pine-cone-shaped heart effectively disappeared some five hundred years ago.

Whilst the heart icon remains firmly anchored in today's visual culture, we are nevertheless witnessing a revival of its naturalistic shape. In modern art, it can be seen, for example, in Nahum Zenil's *Ex-voto* and in Alain Miller's *Eye love eye* (fig.72). It would seem that both painters derived their hearts from an anatomical atlas or from personal observation. The natural heart has also made its return in advertising, an example being the Benetton hearts (fig.73), which are clearly based on reality. That we are witnessing a confrontation between the two shapes, the natural and the icon, is clear from the cover of the CD-ROM in figure 1, where the heart, almost programmatically, is portrayed in both forms.[92]

The question posed by Erwin Panofsky in 1961 will increasingly occur to ordinary mortals as they confront the difference.

ROUGH CHRONOLOGY OF HEART (ICON) SHAPES

Egyptian	Greek	Etruscan Roman Coptic	Medieval	14th Century	15th Century	16th Century	17th Century	18th Century	Modern
heart (urn) and hieroglyph	pine-cone or pyramid shaped	bladder shaped							
	no illustrations								
			Meso-american						
			Ornamental leaves						

The heart as a cave

Hendrik Spiegel's *Antrum Platonicum*

An important representative of the renaissance in the Northern Netherlands was Hendrik Spiegel (fig.76). Born in Amsterdam in 1549, he moved to Haarlem in 1609 and died in Alkmaar in 1612. He came from a wealthy Amsterdam merchant family and held a number of prominent social positions. The author of the first

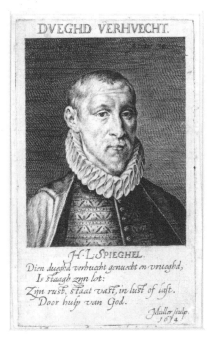

Fig.76. J. Muller, portrait of Hendrik Spiegel, dated 1614.

Dutch grammar, he played a leading role in the movement for the purification and wider use of the Dutch language. His circle of friends included writers and scholars – Roemer Visscher in Amsterdam, Dirck Coornhert in Haarlem, Jan van Hout, Joseph Scaliger, Justus Lipsius and Janus Douza in Leyden – as well as artists like Cornelis Cornelisz, Jan Saenredam and Hendrick Goltzius. Through these contacts, he exerted a pervasive influence on, among others, the young Pieter Cornelisz Hooft and Karel van Mander. His greatest work is *Hertspiegel* ('Heart-mirror'), a long, allegorical poem written in hexameters, in which he set out his non-biblical moral philosophy in a direct though somewhat rambling style. His strong religious faith was based on an amalgamation of Christian, neoplatonic and neostoic ideas, together with an underlying pantheism that sees God manifested in all things.[94]

Hertspiegel has been called the 'first impressive poem of the Northern Dutch renaissance', 'the first comprehensive Dutch poem of modern times' and 'the most important literary accomplishment of the generation before 1600'. Consisting of seven books, it was written between 1577 and 1612, but only published posthumously, in 1614. It is the account of a prolonged introspection on the relationship between Virtue and Happiness: how man can live virtuously on the basis of a rational view of life, keeping emotions, instincts and desires in check, in order to successfully strive to attain God, Truth and Virtue. Although the basis was the Bible, self-analysis, self-education and self-discipline played an important part in Spiegel's ethical system. His personal motto, appearing countless times in his work, summed up his philosophy in two words: *Dueghd verhuecht*, Virtue delights.[95]

Much has been written about Spiegel's literary oeuvre. This essay, however, deals with a relatively unknown aspect: his interest in art. We know that he owned paintings and that, perhaps inspired by similar descriptions in Erasmus, his literary work includes descriptions of imaginary paintings. As we shall see, he also played an active, even initiating, role in the creation of several real works of art. A case in point is the *Antrum Platonicum* (Plato's cave), an engraving by his friend Jan Saenredam (fig.77). It shows a cave divided by a wall,

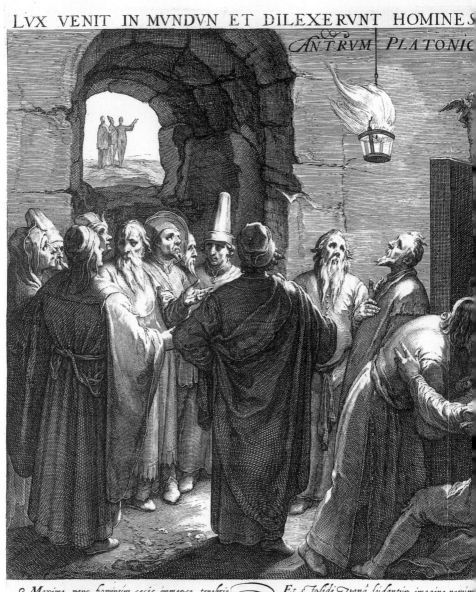

Fig. 77. *Antrum Platonicum*, engraving by Jan Saenredam, 1604, second state.

VM.

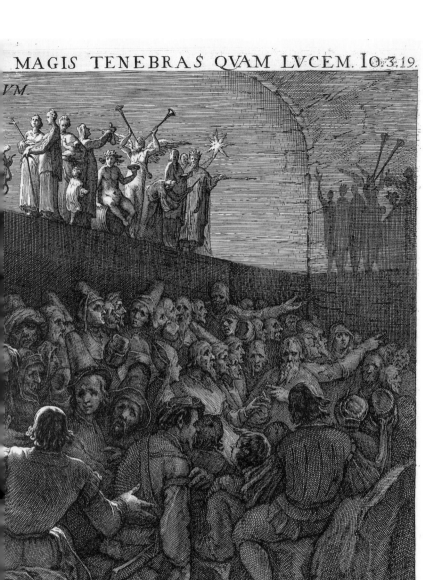

Hi positâ erroris nebulâ dignoscere possunt
Vera bona, atque alios cecâ sub noc̄te latentes
Extrahere in claram lucem conantur, at illis
Nullus amor lucis, tanta es̄ rationis egestas.

C.C. Harlemensis Inv.
Sanredam Sculpsit.
Henr. Hondius excudit.
1604.

Z.D.PET.PAAW IN LVGDVN. ACAD. PROFESSORI MEDICO D.D.

with both areas full of people. On the left is a tunnel leading outside, and a blazing lamp hangs from the ceiling. On the wall are allegorical figures whose shadows are projected onto the opposite wall.[96]

The engraving, dated 1604, was based on a painting by Cornelis Cornelisz of Haarlem, which, although now lost, was described in Karel van Mander's *Grondt der edel vry schilder-const*, published in 1603. Van Mander refers to two famous contemporary Haarlem painters, Cornelis Cornelisz and Hendrick Goltzius. Speaking of the former, he wrote:

> *Plato's cave*, an extremely artful painting by this painter, is in Amsterdam. It is full of reflections of light. A group of captives in the gloom are quarrelling about shadows of figures produced by the light of the lantern. Several of the free inhabitants of the cave can see both the figures and their shadows. In the distance are people looking up into the sky. Let the owner explain what this means.[97]

On Saenredam's print, Cornelisz is given credit as inventor, but the caption *H.L. spiegel figurari et sculpi cvravit. ac Doctissimo ornatissimo qz D.PET.PAAW in Lvgdvn. Acad. Professori Medico D.D.* indicates that Spiegel, and not Cornelisz, was responsible for the idea behind the representation. A passage from the third book of the *Hertspiegel* lends support to this assumption. During a stroll, the poet is taken unawares by a sudden change in the weather; it grows dark, the wind comes up, and beneath his feet the ground opens up, revealing the narrow entrance to a cave:

> It was shaped like a heart. In the twilight I saw a large number of people talking among themselves. One group sat with their backs to a lantern and looked at the opposing wall, on which silhouettes were moving. One looked in

fascination at the shadows of gold and silver coins, another looked in delight at the shadows of pies and pastries. Yet another cast envious glances at a sumptuous crown and sceptre, or at naked Venus, a laurel wreath or a peacock's tail. And as they looked, they made fun of the preferences of the others. Scarcely anyone was giving any thought to his human condition. If such was done, the person concerned would walk over the section on the other side of the wall. There he could see the figures, whom, thus far, he had looked at merely as shadows. Here too people were arguing among themselves. Each preferred the figure on the wall whose shadow he had preferred before. Occasionally, a solitary being would detach itself from the group and retreat from the gloomy cave along the narrow passage leading to the reality of the daylight without. There, a mere handful of souls is gathered. These fortunate beings are not governed by their instincts; with an air of tranquil contentment, they are enjoying the stirrings of their heart.

I enquired of a roughly built, thick-lipped hunch-back what it all signified. He responded by saying that the cave denotes the human heart. The light of the lantern is the ignorance with which everyone begins life. If man remains in this stage, he is tormented by the fear of losing what he has. The shadows regarded so intently signify semblance that makes fools anxious: wealth, status, fame, lechery, arrogance, and so on. Each person prefers his own choice to those of the others, and that is why they are permanently quarrelling. But the satisfaction of desire is only temporary; happiness is not to be found in possessions or sensual stimulation. The thirst for purity of soul, for God, truth and genuine virtue is the true nourishment of the soul.[98]

If frequency of citation of an owner in Van Mander's *Schilder-boeck* is taken as a measure of the size of that person's collection, then Spiegel should be regarded as one of the more important of the Amsterdam collectors. We have seen that Cornelisz' painting was in Amsterdam at the time Van Mander wrote the *Grondt*. A year later he mentions another painting by Cornelisz, *First world or golden age*, in his *Schilder-boeck* (1604). According to Van Mander, the work was 'in the possession of the connoisseur Hendrick Louwersz Spieghel'. In another passage, he refers to 'the art-loving Mr Hendrick Louwersz. Spieghel in Amsterdam'. Considering that Spiegel was well known for his interest in art, that he owned at least one painting by Cornelisz, and taking into account Spiegel's repeated references to Plato's cave, we may assume that Cornelisz' original *Speloncke Platonis* (Plato's cave) was also in Spiegel's possession.[99]

It was the practice of Cornelisz not to sketch his designs for engravings, but to paint them roughly in a few colours on panel. They were executed on the same scale as the print that was to be made. The painting of Plato's cave was thus probably not meant to be an autonomous work of art, but a design for the engraver, and thus a stage in the realization of the intended final product. Apart from Spiegel's dedication of the engraving to his nephew, the Leyden physician Pieter Paaw (1567-1617, fig.78), the detailed description of Plato's cave in the *Hertspiegel* justifies the conclusion that he had initially commissioned Cornelisz to paint, and later had Jan Saenredam engrave, his conception. The painting can be dated circa 1602.[100]

PLATO'S CAVE

In the seventh book of the *Hertspiegel*, written after 1602, the author again refers to Plato's cave, this time to an imaginary painting of it. The poet takes us for a walk along the Amstel river to the isolated country house,

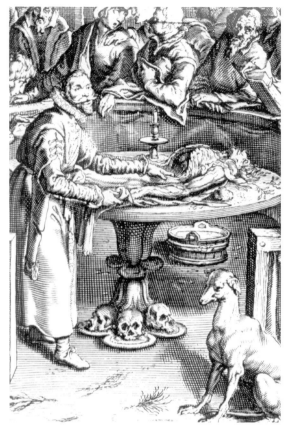

Fig.78. Pieter Paaw, engraving by A.J. Stockius after J. de Gheyn II, 1616.

Ruyschestein. In Spiegel's day, this was the only large such residence on the banks the river; it was situated upstream from the main bend in the Amstel to the south of Amsterdam. He leads us into a hall where Apollo is feasting. Euterpe's organ, closed by two panels like a triptych, is standing against one of the walls. The front is decorated with a painting of Arion on a dolphin, an image which could be described as Spiegel's personal emblem. We may assume that he owned a painting with this scene, also of his own conception, which was painted by Cornelisz and engraved (about 1590) by Jan Muller (fig.79). The print bears Spiegel's personal motto *Dueghd verhuecht*.[101]

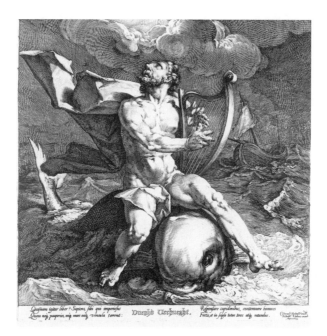

Fig.79. *Arion*, engraving by Jan Muller, probably after a painting by Cornelis Cornelisz, about 1590.

The story of Arion is well known from Greek and Latin literature. The Greek lyre-player from Methymna on the island of Lesbos was invited to a musical contest in Tainaros, Sicily, and was awarded the first prize. With numerous gifts from his admirers, he sailed back to Corinth. But the crew, wanting to get their hands on his money, decided to throw him overboard. When Arion heard of the plan, he offered his possessions in exchange for his life. He was allowed to sing one last time and then to jump overboard. Ceremoniously dressed, he sang an aria and then leapt into the sea with his lyre. However, his singing had attracted a school of dolphins and he was borne on the back of one of them to the harbour of Corinth.

For Spiegel, Arion's rescue by the dolphins signified that it is best to seek virtue by trusting in God. Arion was the personification of that perfect trust. Spiegel's interpretation of the story and the four lines of verse beneath his Arion print are derived from an epigram in Alciati's

Emblematum liber (1531, fig.80). The figure of Arion embodied Spiegel's own personal ideal; he wanted to be the Arion of Amsterdam. Indeed, as he enters the hall in Ruyschestein, he is addressed in song by Euterpe, as if he

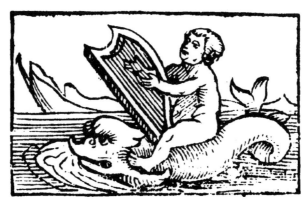

Fig.80. *Arion* from Andrea Alciati, *Emblematum liber*, 1531.

were Arion himself. (As a matter of fact, Arion's face on Muller's print resembles Spiegel. Perhaps it is a portrait of him.)[102]

The panels of Euterpe's organ are opened to reveal a painting of Plato's cave on the inside of one of them:

Behold Plato's cave, in which people argue about idle and senseless matters. Alas, how few people follow Christ without being diverted by earthly images. Most of them cling to the misunderstanding and remain enthralled by the promises that the shadows hold. The proclamation of salvation does not touch them in their heart; they believe in gossip and in the importance of money, luxuriousness, honour and status. Then the organ panels were opened. On the inside of one panel was a painting of Plato's cave, in which man behaves like an animal under the influence of the seductive shadow figures.[103]

It is clear that the allegory of Plato's cave was a favourite theme of Spiegel. In a letter of 16 October 1606 to Pieter Paaw, his eldest sister's son, setting out his ethical views, Spiegel uses the term 'Platoos spelonk' (Plato's cave) as a reference to an allegory which he knew his nephew would understand in all its implications:

> Sweet and soft must she [Virtue] be by nature; but Plato's cave, mistaken reason and [bad] habit stand in her way.

Paaw was indeed aware of the extensive allegorical significance Spiegel attached to this term, he had read the *Hertspiegel* (to which Spiegel also refers in the same letter) and knew Saenredam's engraving and the text accompanying it, which his uncle had dedicated to him two years previously. Let us now consider this representation.[104]

The scene represents a rather free illustration of a passage from Plato's *Republic*. At the beginning of Book seven, Plato describes a group of men who live in a subterranean cave with a long passage opening to the light along its entire width. From childhood, they have had their legs and necks fettered, so that they have had to remain in the same spot and can only look forward, the shackles preventing them from turning their heads. Higher up and at a distance behind them there burns a light. Between the light and these prisoners a road runs above, along which a low wall has been built, similar to the partition separating the public from the exhibitor in puppet shows. Human images, shapes of animals and implements of all kinds pass along the wall. Except for the shadows cast by the light on the cave wall facing them, the cave-dwellers can see neither themselves nor each other. As they speak, they assume that the forms they recognize are the passing objects; to them reality is nothing but the shadows cast by the objects.

In contradistinction to Plato's description, the individuals portrayed in Saenredam's engraving are not shackled. As a substitute for the low puppet-show-like stage, we see a high wall; the lamp behind them casts their shadows on the right wall of a wedge-shaped cave. In the right chamber, we see many men and a few women of every class and age, apparently in the midst of active discussion or argumentation. Another group stands in the left chamber. Instead of the wide passageway described by Plato, we see an exit in the form of a long and narrow tunnel.[105]

Saenredam's engraving has been considered, quite wrongly, to be an illustration for the *Hertspiegel*. Its very size makes this improbable, since the dimensions of the print (27.2 x 44.4 cm) would have required an exceptionally large book. Apart from this, as has been said, the *Hertspiegel* was not published during Spiegel's lifetime; the first edition appeared in 1614 and contained no illustrations. In his preface, the Amsterdam publisher Cornelis Cooll, promised that the second edition would be accompanied by illustrations and annotations, but that too remained unillustrated. In fact, it was the fourth edition, published in Amsterdam in 1694 by Hendrik Wetstein, which was first to contain a copy of the print. It measured roughly half the size of the original.

The *Antrum Platonicum* represents a separate work of art conceived by Spiegel. His ethical views, so extensively elaborated in the *Hertspiegel*, are succinctly and fully summarized in this image. The work has the structure of an emblem. Its motto is a text from the gospel of Saint John 3,19: *Lvx venit in mundun* [sic] *et dilexervnt homines magis tenebras qvam lvcem* [Light is come into the world, and men loved darkness rather than light]. The twelve-line poem below the print serves as the epigram of the emblem and significantly combines the motto and the image, disclosing its symbolic content. While probably no more than a few manuscripts of the *Hertspiegel* existed during his lifetime, Spiegel published the *Antrum* print and distributed it among his friends. It seems only natural that he should have dedicated it to his nephew, Pieter Paaw, with whom he was accustomed to discuss ethical problems, and who had become his closest friend following the death of Dirck Coornhert in 1590.[106]

THE SHAPE OF THE HUMAN HEART

In his dissertation on the *Hertspiegel*, Jong pointed to a remarkable discrepancy, not only between the original description of the cave by Plato and its representation in the engraving of the *Antrum Platonicum*, but also between this print and Spiegel's description of it in Book three of the *Hertspiegel*. The inconsistency lies in the fact that, although he explicitly states on three occasions that the cave is shaped like a human heart, this is not corroborated in the print. Knipping also pointed to this difference. He believed that Spiegel certainly would have preferred the *Antrum* to have had the shape of a heart, as he wrote in the *Hertspiegel*. However, according to Knipping, it is conceivable that the form of the heart was never realized in the engraving either because of the technical inability of the engraver, or because of Spiegel's unwillingness (with respect to Plato) to stretch the point too far. We shall see, however, that the likeness has been overlooked: the cave represented in the engraving does indeed have the internal structure of the heart, as it had been conceived by anatomists since antiquity.[107]

The acquisition of anatomical data would not have been difficult for Spiegel, since Paaw was a well-known physician who had studied at universities in France, Denmark, Germany and Italy. He acquired his anatomical knowledge at the university of Padua, where the father of modern anatomy, Andreas Vesalius, author of the famous *Fabrica*, had taught anatomy in the 1540s. In 1589, Paaw became the first professor of anatomy at Leyden university. His correspondence shows that he had a strong interest in a variety of scientific and artistic subjects. He published commentaries on the works of Hippocrates and Galen, and his fame as an anatomist is shown by a number of prints depicting his public dissections, as well as his anatomical theatre. One of his students, Nicolaas Tulp, a famous physician and anatomist in his own right, has been immortalized in Rembrandt's *Anatomy of Dr. Nicolaas Tulp*.[108]

From Paaw's books on anatomy, it is clear that he was well acquainted with the works of earlier writers. In addition to making use of the *Fabrica* as a handbook, he taught from Vesalius' *Epitome*, which not only provided a descriptive anatomy and an anatomical atlas, but also embodied the principles of his educational method in a more striking fashion than the *Fabrica*. As a matter of fact, Paaw had published an edition of the *Epitome* with extensive comments. In the fourth chapter of this book, concerning the heart, its form is compared to that of a pine-cone containing two chambers. They are like the rooms in which human life is played out. The right chamber is larger than the left; the valves are situated in the opening of the chambers. The right and left chambers have separate outlets, the pulmonary artery ('arterial vein') and the aorta, respectively. The heart is described as having a muscular wall, thicker on the left than on the right.[109]

This conception of the anatomy of the heart does not differ essentially from that which had been accepted prior to the time of Vesalius. It ultimately derived from the description in one of the Hippocratic writings, dating from the third century BC, and from those by Galen from the second century. The latter's work formed the basis of all discussion of cardiac form and function right down to the seventeenth century and the time of Harvey. Broadly speaking, the Galenic concept of the heart, with only a few modifications, was the knowledge Paaw was able to convey to his uncle. A reconstruction of Galen's circulatory system, in which the movement of the blood in both arteries and veins was regarded as a tidal ebb and flow, is shown in figure 81. The structure of Spiegel's *Antrum* is in complete agreement with the Galenic concept of the form of the heart.[110]

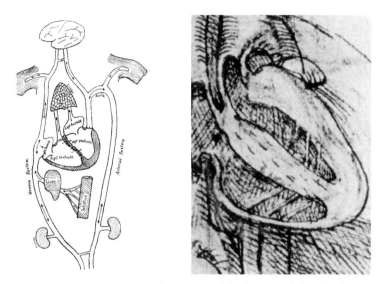

Fig.81. Diagram illustrating Galen's view of the heart and the circulation of the blood, and a cross-section of the heart by Leonardo da Vinci.

In order to illustrate his interpretation of Plato's allegory, Spiegel needed a diagram of the heart, one side of which was to be left open, so that the observer could view its inside obliquely from above. To this end, he omitted the base of the heart. Figure 82 represents a cross-section with the base removed along a line connecting the left wall of the aorta and the middle of the right atrium, then considered to be part of the great vein. An outline of the *Antrum* (fig.83) shows definite agreement with this anatomy, viz. the passage originating from the left chamber corresponds to the aorta. In the lower right corner, a round, concave stone formation corresponding to one of the cardiac valves, the *tricuspid*, is just visible. At this time, the tricuspid valve was described as occupying a position between the great vein (*vena cava*) and the right chamber. In Paaw's words: *cavae venae orificium ad hunc pertinet* (the orifice of the great vein reaches this far). His detailed

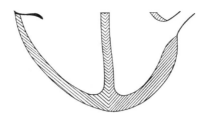

Fig.82. Diagram of Galen's concept of the heart,
according to Paaw's description.

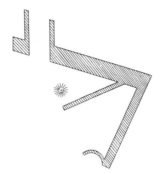

Fig.83. Diagram of Spiegel's *Antrum Platonicum*.

anatomical contribution must have been an additional
reason for Spiegel's dedicating the engraving to him.

The uncle sought the nephew's advice both before
and after the first state of the engraving. This can be seen
from the addition of the far corner to the cave, seen in
the final version of the print (fig.77 on pages 87 and 88).
In the first state (fig.84), the wall of the cave had a
hyperbolic form. In the works of the classical anatomist,
however, specific attention is paid to the position of the
apex, the tip of the heart. Its precise location varies from
one source to another; it is not always clear whether the
apex is a part of the left or the right chamber. This
confusion can be clearly seen in a passage from Galen's
On anatomical procedures: 'the left ventricle [is] extending
to the apex, and the right ending much below it, and
often with an outline of its own'. Avicenna must have
intended to say the same when he wrote that 'the base
of the right cavity descends much lower'.[111]

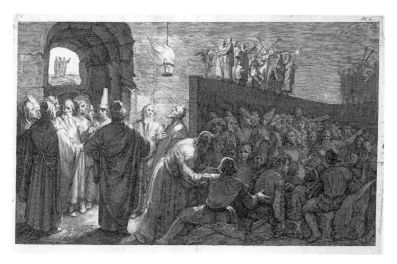

Fig.84. *Antrum Platonicum*, engraving by Jan Saenredam, first state.

All the classical and medieval anatomists were agreed that the right chamber of the heart is larger than the left. That Paaw shared the conviction can be seen from his commentary on Vesalius' *Epitome*, in which he states *horum qui dexter capacior multo sinistro* (the right-hand one of these [i.e. the chambers] is much larger than the left).

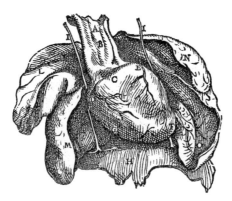

Fig.85. An illustration of the heart from Vesalius' *Fabrica*, 1543. *F* indicates the apex.

As a consequence of this, it seems logical to assume that the lowest point of the cavity is part of the right chamber. In fact, the illustrations found in Vesalius' *Fabrica* (fig.85) also show the apex as a part of the right chamber. Paaw was left with little choice: in order to divide a wedge-shaped space into a large and a smaller section, he was obliged to place the corner of the wedge in the larger space, i.e. the right chamber (fig.83 on page 100).[112]

The *Antrum*, with its 'vulgar' right chamber, its 'aristocratic' left compartment, and the flame leaping in the direction of the tunnel (aorta), gives rise to associations with early as well as contemporary physiological concepts. The flaming lantern in the left compartment of the *Antrum* goes back to classical medical texts. According to the Hippocratic writings, human intelligence, the principle which rules over the soul, is situated in the left chamber. This is where the vital spirit is generated from a source of 'untempered heat'. The heat of the heart is compared with the flame of a burning lamp. This concept was also accepted by Plato, who specifically mentions the fire *(pyr)* in the heart. Aristotle considered the heart the central source of heat, containing the flame of life.[113]

These ideas are also found, with variations, in Galen, who described the left chamber of the heart as the furnace of the vital fire, comparing it to a flaming lamp. In accordance with Galenic teaching, Vesalius explains that in the left ventricle, undoubtedly the most 'noble' half of the heart, the crude blood from the right ventricle, the air from the lungs and the 'innate heat' combine to form blood endowed with *pneuma*, the vital spirit, which is distributed throughout the whole body and serves the higher functions of the organs, which it reaches by way of the 'great artery' (i.e. the aorta, which is represented in the print by the tunnel leading to the outside and towards where the flame is fluttering). The father of modern anatomy carefully explained that, as far as physiology was concerned, he had brought his views into line with Galenic doctrine, because the scope of the *Fabrica* could not permit either enforcing new physiological opinions or swerving 'a nail's breadth from the doctrines of the Prince of medicine'.[114]

The representation of the cave in the print agrees almost exactly with the description in the third book of the *Hertspiegel*. An exception to this are the allegorical figures on the wall, which form a rather random group of eleven virtues and vices (fig.86). Their names are

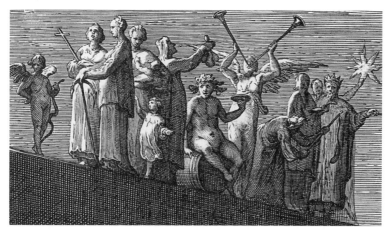

Fig.86. The allegorical figures on the wall in the *Antrum Platonicum*.

regularly mentioned in the *Hertspiegel*, but not as part of a specific group and not in this sequence. The *Antrum* also corresponds to a short summary of its essence in Spiegel's *ABC Kettinglied* (ABC Chain Song), a series of twenty-four quatrains on the alphabet, which have been added to every edition of the *Hertspiegel* since 1615. One of the verses summarizes it as follows:

> Baat-schyn van wellust, faam, gheld, hoghe staten,
> Bekoort elk heil-lust onverzaad te laten
> Inwendigh: om uytwendigh zoeken lust
> in waanghoed, dat ons lyf en ziel ontrust.

(The apparent advantage of luxuriousness, fame, money or status hinders the striving for inner salvation. The search for outer appearance disturbs body and soul).

Some of the virtues and vices are mentioned in the poem, but the text fails to explain the specific constellation of the figures on the wall.

A number of them can easily be identified: the first four are Amor, Fides, Spes and Caritas. According to Augustinian, neoplatonic theory, there is a paradox in the opposition and coincidence of man's love of God and love of himself, the root of Caritas: 'Love thy God, love thy neighbour; God as God, thy neighbour as thyself'. We may assume that the Caritas on the wall stands for love of one's neighbour. Since love of God was the complement of love of one's neighbour, the two forms were really inseparable. A scene typifying *amor proximi* would therefore imply the presence of the other aspect of that virtue, *amor Dei*, divine or pure love. In his voluminous moral treatise published in 1586 at the insistence of Hendrik Spiegel, Dirck Coornhert also distinguishes between eternal and transitory love. Coornhert had illustrated this difference more than ten years before on the title page of *Das Buch Extasis* by Jan van der Noot (fig.87). It shows a triumphal arch and includes a Caritas-like Venus holding a heart and accompanied by Amor. In the foreword of the book, Venus is described as a smiling figure of beauty, thereby inducing virtue in the onlooker. Amor is described as 'the trustee Cupid (lauded by Plato and other poets) who encourages people toward unending divine matters', and who, like 'the burning heart of Venus', represents the love a pious man feels for God and his neighbour. The first and foremost in the row of figures on the wall is thus *Amor divinus*, a role which he had also assumed in emblematics. In an emblem by Gilles Corrozet, Love and Virtue stand like deities on a column (fig.88). Like Caritas, Virtue holds a heart in her right hand. The connection between the two kinds of love is also clearly referred to in the *Hertspiegel*: man owes God 'thanks, praise and love, fraternal love too'. This results in 'purity of heart', the fruits of which, in turn, is love of God above all else.[115]

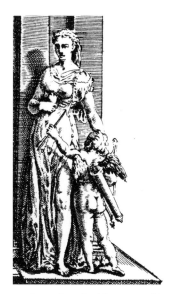

Fig.87. Venus and Amor on Coornhert's title page of *Das Buch Extasis*, ca. 1573.

The fifth figure on the wall, the first of the Vices, is shown facing away from the Virtues. She holds a money-pouch, known at the time as a *stock-beurs* (lit. stick-purse). She stands for Worldliness or Riches and appears as *Diffidentia dei*, i.e. Distrust in God, in the *Prosopographia*

Amour accompagnée de vertu.

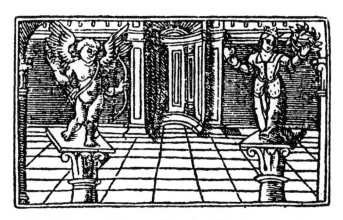

Fig.88. *Love and Virtue*, emblem by Gilles Corrozet 1540.

105

by Philip Galle, a native of Haarlem and a friend of Coornhert and Goltzius (fig.89). In Spiegel's cave, the figure is intended to have a more narrow significance, viz. that of Avarice, who was frequently pictured with a

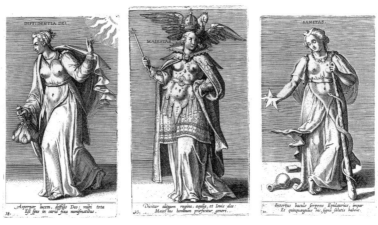

Fig.89. Philip Galle's *Diffidentia dei*, *Maiestas* and *Sanitas*, 1594.

money-pouch as an attribute. Thus, it is not simply coincidental that she has her back turned to Caritas: in the moral teachings of the Church, avaritia is the counterpart of the misericordia aspect of Caritas.[116]

Next on the wall comes Bacchus, symbol of gluttony, seated on a barrel. The figure with two trumpets standing next to him is Fame (Ydele eer, Roemzucht). The figure bending over is wearing a fool's cap. It is holding a stick like a fishing rod, to which a stuffed sausage-shaped object is attached, the fool's bauble (fig.90). The sausage recalls the German *Hans Wurst* (*Hanswurst*) and the Dutch *Hans Worst* (*Hansworst*), a name for a Fool which had already appeared in Sebastian Brant's *Ship of fools* (1494) and in a pamphlet of 1541 authored by Luther.[117]

The next figure, holding an open book, represents False learning ('Schijn-geleerdheid', 'Weetzucht'), the despicable academic knowledge that diverts people from

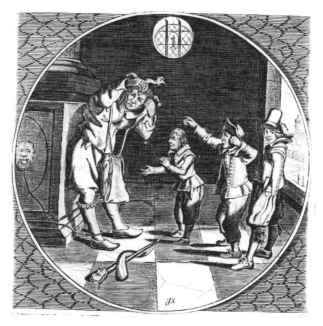

Fig.90. Fool with cap and stuffed sausage-like plaything
attached to the marotte, from Jacob Cats' *Proteus*, 1618.

virtue, and which Spiegel repeatedly and expressly
contrasts with True knowledge ('Heil-geleerdheid' or
'Ware kennis'). Behind this figure stands a king with a
crown and sceptre, symbolizing Majesty or Haughtiness
('Hoge Staat', 'Hoocheid', 'Hovaardy', 'Staat-ziek',
'Pracht-in-Kleed'), terms frequently encountered in the
Hertspiegel. A similar figure also appears in Galle's *Prosopo-
graphia* (fig.89).[118]

The final figure, holding a star, resembles Sanitas
(Health), the figure from Galle's book, who also holds a
star in her hand. The significance of this figure recalls a
passage in the *Hertspiegel* in which the divisions between
the churches are compared to the debates in medical and
other sciences. The 'virtuous' man treats these disputes for
what they are: a well-tended soul ensures the health of the
body. This figure is thus a reference to the preoccupation
with the welfare of the body rather than of the soul.[119]

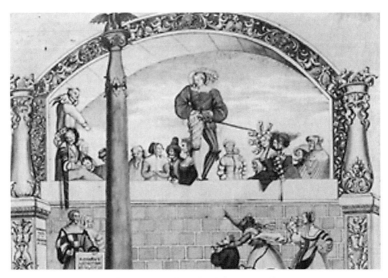
Fig.91. Niklaus Deutsch, *The idolatry of Solomon*, 1518.

The presence of both good and evil characteristics also accords with Galen's concept of the heart as the source of passion, and, of course, with Spiegel's, that, by introspection, man must distinguish between his good and bad tendencies.

The idea of setting figures on a wall was not new in art. A large fresco illustrating the text of 1 Kings 11:1-8 painted on a wall of the house of Antoni Noll in Basle in 1518 shows Solomon being tempted to worship idols (fig.91). One of them is positioned above him on a terrace wall amidst a number of men and women accompanied by negative attributes, as well as idols or vices that look down from this high wall. Noll's house was at the corner of the Muensterplatz and the Kesslergasse. The fresco survived until 1758, so it is possible that Saenredam, Goltzius, Matham or another of Spiegel's friends saw it while journeying to Italy.[120]

In addition to the print's emblematic structure, the fact that the figures on the wall do not correspond in number and order to the vices and virtues referred to in Spiegel's texts further argues for it being an independent work of art.

Its autonomy is also apparent from the slight discrepancy between the interpretation of the allegory in the *Hertspiegel* and the three quatrains, beneath the engraving:

The majority of men wallow forever in the blind darkness which enwraps them, and rejoice in their empty ardour. Look how their eyes cling to the shadows in front of them, how they all admire and love the simulacra of Truth,

and are stupidly fooled by an illusion of reality. Only a few of superior clay, standing apart from the stupid mass in pure light, realise that the shadows of things are all sham and weigh everything with the proper scales.

They are able to break away from the fog of error and to discern the true Good; and they try to draw the others, who hide in a blind night, into the clear light. But these do not love the light at all, so great is their lack of understanding.[121]

The last stanza refers to the two figures in the foreground of the print (they who 'try to draw the others'), attempting to convince those who remain in darkness to come out into the light. The figure leaning forward and trying to get the people in the shadows to repent represents Christ, in accordance with the lesson that Spiegel himself gives to those who spend their lives in darkness: that they may only hope to leave their place through Christ's help. His seated assistant, who is seen from the rear, and acts as an intermediary, appears to be younger. He may represent Saint John the Evangelist, a quotation from whose gospel heads the print.[122]

The attitude of the 'Christ' figure in the print reminds one of his descent into limbo, a scene often represented in the middle ages and the renaissance. He appears at the entrance to a cave, where he rescues the 'righteous'

109

heathen of the Old Testament by breaking open the gateway to the caves at the entrance to hell and liberating the imprisoned souls (fig.92).[123]

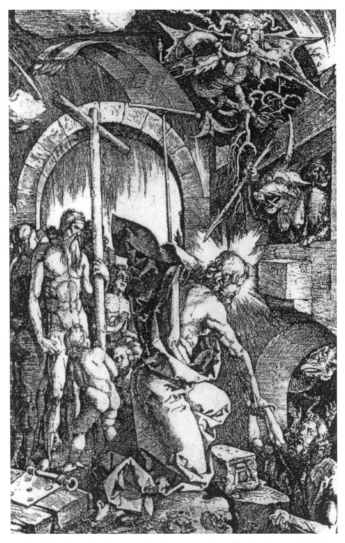

Fig.92. Albrecht Dürer, *Christ descents into limbo*, about 1510.

Two classical allegories dominated Spiegel's philosophy: one was the parable of Plato's cave, the other that of Cebes' *Tabula*, a dialogue in Greek, probably dating from the first century, which, in Spiegel's day, was attributed to Cebes, a pupil of Socrates. The Greek manuscript was discovered in the fifteenth century and first published in 1494. A Latin translation appeared in 1498; the first Dutch translation appeared in 1564 and was followed by many other editions, some illustrated. The dialogue contains an allegory that influenced Spiegel's life and work even more strongly than the allegory of Plato's cave. He started studying Greek when he got older, in order to be able to read Cebes' text in the original. He provided an account of its contents on three occasions: in a full translation, first printed, posthumously, in 1615; in a synopsis, *Kebes tafereels kort begrip*, a free poetic extract, printed together with the translation; and in a paraphrase, which forms an important part of Books six and seven of the *Hertspiegel*. [124]

In the *Tabula,* an old man elucidates the meaning of an allegorical mural in a fictitious temple for the benefit of its visitors. It is a mirror of human life, illustrating the different kinds of human behaviour; virtue and vice play an important part in it. The scene described consists of three terraces arranged, in most of the illustrations, in a tiered structure of three concentric rings. The outermost contains young, inexperienced and ignorant people who are about to embark upon life. They can spend it there in sin and vice, punishment and misery, but to improve their lot, they can also enter the second ring. At its entrance, there stands a beautiful and attractively dressed young woman, Education, but she turns out to be False education or False learning. After a while, one may ascend to the third ring, albeit difficult to reach, by climbing an almost impassable rock. Here is located True education, higher insight into the meaning of life, the road to blessedness, also personified in a female figure.

The finest representation of the *Tabula* in the visual arts is that by Hendrick Goltzius, engraved by his stepson Jacob Matham in 1592, in three large plates, the largest ever made in Goltzius' workshop (fig.93 on page 113). Spiegel must have owned a copy; he may have had this in mind when he described the panels of the fictional organ of Euterpe he came across in Ruyschestein during his poetic stroll along the banks of the Amstel. We have seen that the panels were decorated with two scenes of Spiegel's own invention, *Arion on the dolphin* on the exterior and the *Antrum Platonicum* on the inside of one of them (see page 94). The inside of the other was decorated with a representation of the *Tabula Cebetis*.[125]

Further, in the sixth book of the *Hertspiegel*, the author is awakened by the muse Erato, who starts to change the interior of his small summer house. She fills it with paintings, each conveying a moral message. The entire north wall of the front hall is covered by the *Tabula*, the meaning of which is explained to Spiegel by the muse.[126]

Spiegel's paraphrases of the *Tabula Cebetis* contain valuable information for the iconography of the *Antrum Platonicum*. The major part of these digressions is devoted to the description of the type of individual who can easily be identified in the right chamber of the cavern, in which a number of persons are listening to the expostulations of an old man, while others do not seem to be aware of his presence and are busily talking in separate groups. The 'ordinary man' is enslaved by the mere appearance of things and is eagerly looking for the shadows of Honour, Prestige, Wealth, Sensuality, and whatever he considers to be good.

Seated in the first ring of the *Tabula* is the Nature God, an old, wise man, willing to teach the ways of life to those who will listen. He points out that Selfishness, Intemperance and Sensuality bring forth disastrous fruits, and that False learning does not lead to True knowledge. Those who do not follow this ancient law of

nature continually stumble, lead a wretched life, and, in the long run, are disillusioned. Sickness and health appear at the end of the *Tabula* text: just as a pious death is preferable to a wicked life, sickness is sometimes preferable to good health. This reminds us of the presence of Sanitas as the final figure on the wall in the *Antrum*.[127]

In the second ring of the *Tabula,* there are individuals of a different type who, although they have become aware of their former, primitive errors through reflection, maintain that they can fulfil their needs by False knowledge. These people encounter a number of vices in female form, the enumeration of which, more than any other of the vices in the *Hertspiegel*, brings to mind the figures standing on the wall in the *Antrum*:

> Most of them remain corrupted in their heart, full of errors, without pride; greedy and lustful, vain, ambitious, slothful, malicious, envious and mean. But they are, above all, conceited and haughty, and look down on all those who love the things of nature instead of repeating the words of the learned.[128]

The individuals of the second ring are the merely pseudo-learned. Cebes sums them up: poets, orators, dialecticians, mathematicians, geometers, astrologers, Epicureans, critics, and so on. In his *Tabula* synopsis, Spiegel refers to them as ten types of temporary or permanent residents. Seven of the ten are engaged in the arts; they correspond to the seven liberal arts: poets, orators, dialecticians, musicians, mathematicians, geometers and astronomers. The remaining three are different kinds of philosophers: Epicureans, Stoics and Academics.[129]

These pseudo-learned of the *Tabula* must have been the model for the learned in the left chamber of the *Antrum*. None of them discovers the narrow passage leading to the outside world. Most of them stand with their backs to the exit, and all are looking either at the lamp or at the figures on the wall. They show no interest in the shadows, but concentrate on Honour, Prestige and Fame. One standing in the left foreground looks like the female figure who represents False Education. She wears slippers, marking her off from the men, and her headware is feminine too. She matches the description in the *Tabula*: 'at the entrance stands a woman who appears to be altogether pure and neatly adorned'. Her raised arm indicates that she is speaking. She also brings to mind the passage in which Spiegel describes the figure of False Education from the *Tabula*, but in more negative terms:

> Ziett daar voort tweede park een schoone vrouw, die reijnlijk, en cierlijk is gekleet; Dees noemtmen algemeijnlijk Geleertheijt, want zij maakt den menschen school-geleert.

> (Behold in the second ring a beautiful woman who is dressed neatly and elegantly. Everyone calls her Education, but she confers mere textbook learning on mortals.)

The same female figure, Fucata eruditio, stands beside the entrance to the second ring in Goltzius' *Tabula*. She is teaching from a book.[130]

One may wonder whether the man with the halo-like hat, the centre of which is exactly aligned to the vertical middle line of the entrance to the tunnel, is a portrait of Spiegel. His features somewhat resemble those of Arion on the dolphin (fig.94, see also fig.79 on page 93). A male figure sitting in the shadowy right-hand chamber with a similar halo-like brim to his hat also looks like Spiegel. He is one of the two men who have noticed the presence of Christ and have turned away from the silhouettes on the wall.[131]

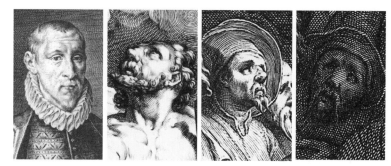

Fig.94. Portraits of H.L. Spiegel, at the age of 30 in 1579, as Arion at the age of 41 in 1590, at the age of 55 in 1604, as one of the philosophers in the left chamber of the *Antrum Platonicum*, and as one of the unenlightened in the dark chamber of the *Antrum*.

The third type of individual, who acquires True knowledge, by conquering False education, walks in the light of truth. In the *Tabula*, this type of individual reaches the highest level by way of a steep and narrow path that only very few tread. At the end of it stand two women, radiant and healthy in body, who are 'eagerly stretching forth their hands'. They are encouraging a third figure, who is being shown the way to the right path. The narrow pathway to the light is not mentioned directly in Spiegel's paraphrases, but this element is clearly present in his *Antrum*. The three female figures on the hillock outside the cave correspond to the virtues on the top of the mountain, the 'Domicilium salutis', of the *Tabula*.

Plato's cave allegory is in agreement with that of the *Tabula Cebetis* as interpreted by Spiegel: deception and misunderstanding are the root of all evil. Both allegories illustrate the path of man's spiritual development. The morphological characteristics of the cavern exactly coincide with the internal structure of the heart, but also, certain details, necessary for Spiegel's cave allegory (virtues and vices on the wall, the lamp), fit in remarkably well with the heart, standing for the seat of the soul, emotions and the flame of life. The narrow exit fulfils the requirements of both the symbolism and Cebes' allegory. The wide opening which Plato described for his cave has been replaced by a narrow tunnel, thereby strengthening the analogy with anatomy, as well as with its symbolic meaning.[132]

Spiegel and Goltzius must have seen earlier representations of the *Tabula*; numerous versions were produced in the sixteenth century in Frankfurt, Vienna, Cracow, Venice, Paris and elsewhere. There are two Northern Netherlandish paintings in Cassel from the second half of the sixteenth century that recall the *Tabula* - *Antrum* pendants of the triptych on Euterpe's organ. One of them is of the *Tabula*, the other is of an enormous cave with two exits (figs. 95 and 96). Inside the second one is the underworld, as described by Virgil in the sixth

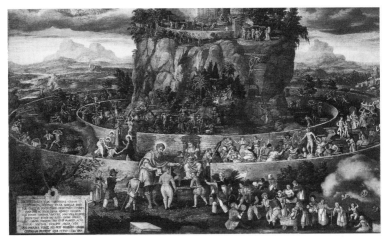

Fig.95. *Tabula Cebetis*, Northern Netherlands, second half of the 16th century.

book of the *Aeneid*. Spiegel may have seen these exceptional pendants, but for those on Euterpe's organ, he may have preferred the cave of his much admired Plato to the scene of Virgil's underworld, which was less appropriate for his ethical message.[133]

The hunchback outside Plato's cave in the *Antrum* passage of the *Hertspiegel* who is asked by the poet to explain the scene (see the paraphrased passage on page 90), can

118

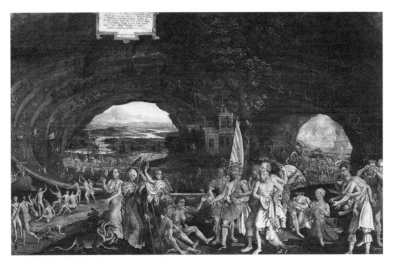

Fig.96. Virgil's *Underworld*, counterpart to figure 95, Northern Netherlands, second half of the 16th century.

be identified as Socrates. In the *Hertspiegel,* he is mentioned more frequently than any other philosopher as a teacher and is even placed on the same footing as Christ. It was only natural to assign him the role of explaining the deeper meaning of Plato's *Antrum,* since he was the source for the allegory of the cave in the *Republic.* Besides, he had played the same role as the inventor of that other classical ethical allegory, the *Tabula,* for this work was regarded as a Socratic dialogue too. The hunchbacked Socrates already appeared on an earlier print of the *Tabula,* in which he is also situated outside the frame of the scene (fig.97).[134]

Spiegel assumed a similar role. When Erato appears to him in a dream in the sixth book of the *Hertspiegel,* he cites Socrates and projects the scene of the *Tabula* onto the wall of his room. He also created his own variant of it by projecting an ethical content similar to that of the *Tabula* onto the interior of the heart-shaped Platonic (Socratic) cave.

119

There was another, less well-known, representation that contributed to Spiegel's conception of the heart-shaped cave: a large-scale didactic print issued in Cologne by Niclas Bombarghen (fig.98). He was printer to Hendrick Niclaes, founder and father of the heretical (liberal) Christian sect known as the House of love (later in England called the *Family of love*). His voluminous theological work *Den spegel der gherechticheit* (The mirror of justice) was published by Christopher Plantin (another member of the sect) between 1535 and 1560. Various works by Niclaes were translated into English in the 1570s and thus influenced the Quakers and John Bunyan's *Pilgrim's progress* and *Holy war*. The Dutch sympathisers with the House of love often held influential positions, and Niclaes was personally acquainted with Spiegel's circle, including Coornhert, Goltzius and Lipsius. Spiegel must have been well informed about the ethical publications and visual expressions of Hendrick Niclaes and his co-believers.[135]

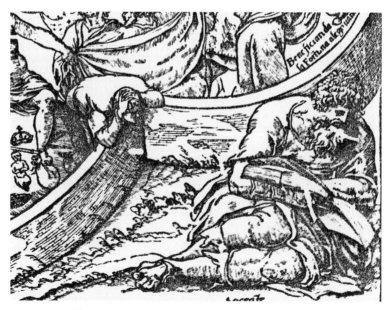

Fig.97 Socrates in a Venetian *Tabula Cebetis*, about 1565.

The invention of this print is attributed to Niclaes himself on the basis of the motto it contains, *Caritas extorsit*. The composition is heart-shaped and represents 'The fall of man and his progress and his return'. Beneath this title are two quotations from the gospels: 'Because strait is the gate, and narrow is the way, which leadeth unto life, and few there be that find it' (Matthew 7:14), and 'Strive to enter in at the strait gate: for many, I say unto you, will seek to enter in, and shall not be able' (Luke 13:24).

Its centre is occupied by the Fall of Adam and Eve. From this point on, the righteous man, armed with a shield bearing the word *Hoop* (Hope), proceeds as a skeleton. On his journey through life, he is accompanied by an allegorical warrior Intelligence (*Gedachten*) armed with the Sword of the spirit (*Zwaard van de geest*). They avoid the vice-filled forest and pass by a circular wall that recalls the walls around the rings of the *Tabula Cebetis*. In both scenarios, man is constrained by all kinds of temptations and vices. In the end, he passes through a narrow passage, like those in the *Tabula* and in the *Antrum*, in this case into the forest of virtues; then he reaches the Tree of God (*Boom van God*), beside which are standing a man and a woman who symbolize the 'new man' who has been freed by Truth.

Niclaes may have borrowed the idea of depicting the path man takes on earth within the outline of a heart icon from the 'cordiform maps' which originated in the course of the sixteenth century. Their longest dimension was longitudinal, the shortest across the parallels. The North pole lay in its upper, concave part, the South pole on its opposite, pointed extremity. At least eighteen of these heart icon-shaped world maps featured in various geographical atlases published between 1511 and 1566. An example is the general map by Johannes Honterius (fig.99).[136]

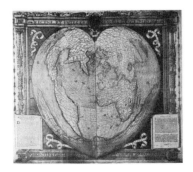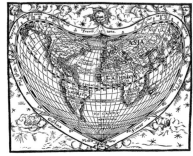

Fig.99. Cordiform world maps by Oronce Fine, 1534, and Johannes Honter, 1561.

SPIEGEL'S SYNTHESIS

It is clear that Niclaes' print has given shape to an ethical narrative like that of the *Tabula* within the contour of a heart. After him, and undoubtedly influenced by this print, Spiegel situated a similar ethical allegory in Plato's cave. All these ingredients – the cave, the *Tabula* and the Heart of love – already existed and were related to one another. What Spiegel achieved in his *Antrum* was a synthesis of them.

The vast number of meanings Spiegel ascribed to the heart should be borne in mind. The heart, the centre of man in Stoic philosophy, was the central symbol in his life. There is scarcely a page in his writings in which the word 'heart' or a compound form does not appear. The *Hertspiegel* itself is a multilayered humanistic pun. Translated literally, it means 'the mirror of the heart'. On the other hand, it can be read as 'Spiegel's heart', an account of what goes on in his heart, and that, as he writes at the beginning of his first book, is of the most service to himself. In that sense, the title can be parsed as 'the mirror of the heart of Spiegel'. In this respect, he was followed by his older friend Coornhert, who shared his preoccupation with ethical and religious matters. The second syllable of Coornhert's name is the Dutch for 'heart'. In 1589, years after Spiegel had begun his magnum opus, Coornhert wrote an ethical work also

called *Hert-spiegel*, which can be taken to mean 'mirror of Coornhert's heart'.[137]

The *Hertspiegel* is an egotistic work of art, a dissertation on the writer's view of life, and, at the same time, a mystical, sometimes even esoteric, monologue. Although throughout his life, he followed an Erasmian-style catholicism, Spiegel was a typical neoplatonic rationalist whose ethics were based on the necessity of knowing one's self and on the assumption that human nature is essentially good. Reason is the guiding principle of life and must control earthly desires. This is only possible if one has learned to distinguish salvation from false salvation and truth from illusion. The hunchback concludes his description of the *Antrum* with this significant moral advice:

Ghi Spiegel, spiegelt u, u heil zoekt int bewerken.

(Thou Spiegel, mirror thyself, work on thyself for thy salvation.)[138]

Spiegel's *Antrum* is his personal version of the *Tabula Cebetis* and remains one of the most remarkable contributions to the symbolism of the heart. Karel van Mander must have been aware of the allegorical significance of the concept, as evidenced by the line with which, tongue in cheek, he rather abruptly concludes his description of Cornelisz' painting: 'den sin beveel ick die 't stuck is eyghen'. This sentence was translated (incorrectly) by Hoecker as: 'The meaning of the work I leave entirely in the hands of the inventor' ('Den Sinn des Werkes überlasse ich dem, welcher das Stück erfunden hat'). This translation would seem to imply that the inventor of the representation was someone other than the painter. However, two (correct) interpretations are possible: 'The meaning of the work I entrust to its owner'; but also: 'The meaning of the work I leave to those who understand it'.[139]

APPENDICES

APPENDIX 1
Van Mander, *Grondt* 7, 45, fol. 32v, 33r.

D'een is te recht een Schilder, van den gonen
Is t'Amsterdam de Speloncke *Platonis*,
In welcke dat Conste meer als ghewoon is.
Daer sietmen Reflexy over al schampen,
Doch een hoop ghevanghen in 't doncker laghen,
Die met Argumenten schenen te campen,
Van Beelde-schaduwen door 't licht der Lampen,
Eenighe los, beelden en schaduw saghen,
Ander verder van daer hadden gheslaghen
Diep in den Hemel t' ghesicht, sonder neyghen,
Maer den sin beveel ick die t' stuck is eyghen.

APPENDIX 2
Hertspiegel 3. 71-135, Veenstra 68-71.

en voor mijn voeten barst een hollen-aarden spleet,
afbreukich engh den ingangh, onder vlak, en breet;
Van maxel was dit hol eens menschen hert geleken
vol volx in scheemrinch licht, diens woord-rijk twistich spreken
als een gemommeldons mij eerst in d'ooren scheen,
dies schoor-voets deijzed' ik nieus-gierich na beneen
in t' twist-hol schaduw-rijk vol trotzich waan-vermeeten
zach ik ontelbre menschen ruggelings gezeten
na t'flonker-fakkel-licht dat zon, en maan verbrant;
Elk staar-ooght nechtigh op een voorgestelde want,
daar beurt-wijs schaduw-beelds vast allerleij vertieren,
die lieft elk zonderlingh na lust, of erf-manieren:
D'een loert versuft op goutt, en silver-schijfkens rondt,
d'aar guwt, naer schaduw-taart en vlâe met open mont:
zulk lonkt na valsche kroon, en schepters maxel heerlijk;
Die loerooght op den schauw des naakten Venus geerlijk:
Dees Faam-ziek steelwijs gluijrt na d'opper lauwer-krans;
Ant' trage eezels beelt hanght d'aar zijn zinnen gansch;

127

Der Pauwen staart-gepraal zulk ander mint hovaardich;
En meenich lieft verzott een gulzich swijn onaardich;
Dees wolven bloedich prijst; die leeuwen, Beeren fel;
Elk schept beangste vreucht in schauw-beelds apen-spel.
Op t'pluijm-rijk veder-bos, op paarden, honden, bloemen,
onwaardich schaduw goett, ondoenlijk al te noemen,
bezonder zonderlingh ziet ellik nijver op
en prijst met anders smaat hoogh zijn gekooren pop
tott kijf, Ia vechtens toe: maar wil hen ijmant straffen
als honden kregel-bits zij meest al tegens blaffen.
zeer zelden ijmant daar op ziel-bezinningh acht,
of beurtet somwijl, flux wert die leer-gier gebracht
te rugh, verbij een muijr die hij de rugh toe keerde,
daar beelden (welker schauw hij eerst voor al begeerde)
gedraghen worden, die hij dan voor schauw-spel prijst;
Doch twist, en onrust mee bij beelde-minnaars rijst.
verwaant, halsstarrich, want elk lieft daar even nechtigh
de beeld-kund, als hij voormaals hingh an schauw-min pleghtig.
En bij dees kleijnen hoop heeft heijl-leer kleijn gehoor
het is zoo t'was; elk waant ook dat hij t'best heeft voor,
En zelden, immer zelden dees van beeld-liefd scheijden
om uijt (door hert hols enghte) zich te laten leijden
van lamp-lichts schaduw-beelds; van t'donker valsch gesicht
tot warer dinghen toon in t'Godlijk zonnen licht;
derwaarts ik zach, en rees daar wel bedaarde menschen
genooten stille vreucht na al haar herten wenschen.
k'anrand' een dik-lip grof, wanschapen, hoogh-gebult
na groett, en weder-groett, hebdij kund, tijt, gedult,
berecht mij (zeijd' ik) wat dees hol-twist is te zeggen,
dees beeld, en schaduw-liefd. Hij gingt aldus uijtleggen.
      T'hol is een ijders hert; het lamp-licht ijdel waan
die ellik eerst ontmoett; blijft hij daar stip op staan,
hem plaaght onrustich leedt, door ijdel- liefds behaghen;
moet niet na droom-vangsts waan aardthaijl-lusts honger plagen?
De schauw-beelds die ghij hem anschouwen ziet met lust
is t'schijn-goedt valsch dat d'achteloosen al ontrust,
als rijkdom, hooghe staat, faam, wellust, weetsucht prachtigh,
en zulke ijlheijd meer; daar menschen onaandachtich
recht als hun hooghste goett partijdich hert, en zin
opstellen; dit maakt twist. Wie eenich lust-gewin

128

verkrijgt, verblijt een tijdt: Dewijl doch wankelbaarlijk
het blijven is, zoo valt verlies, of vrees beswaarlijk
dien, die of zoekt, of lieft zulk waan-goett onbedocht.
Maar of Fortuijns onsta daar iemant oijt bezocht?
die vint niet lijkewel in valsch goett waar genoeghen
hem prikkelt onderwijl zijn ziel-heijl-hongers wroeghen:
Godt, waarhcijt, waarc dcuchdt is onser zielen spijs.
vergeefs el zoeken menschen reukeloos, onwijs
in schauw-lust haar genoecht. kan schijn t'gemoett vermaken
geduijrich? en of zij tott beelde-kennis raaken,
leijt die niet tott de daad, z'ist maar een valsche stutt;
beeld-kennis daadeloos, als schauw-kun blijft onnutt.
Waarschijnlijk vande deuchd veel treffelijk kunnen spreken;
ja lokken andren aan door haar boet-vaardich preeken;
Maar zoo ghij al haar doen, en leeven wel besseft,
de daat zeijt klapping-kunst haar zellefs hert niet treft.
Ghij Spieghel spiegelt u, u heijl zoekt in t'bewerken

APPENDIX 3
Hertspiegel 7. 89-99, Veenstra 178-179.

ziett hier in Platoos hol, qua anwenst, ijdel wenschen,
en twist om schijn-goett valsch: Helaas; Hoe luttel menschen
zich, en der dinghen heijl door reen-wiks hulp slaan gae,
veel min gansch beeld, en wille-loos Christ volghen nae;
qua voor-gangh, mis-verstands anwenst houtt u gebonden
aan schaduw-heijls onrust; Dies waarheijts heijl verkonden
u niett ter herten raakt; of lòòft ment met de praat,
men lòòft in s'hertsen gront gelt, wellust, eer en staat:
Mits gingh de Orghel op: An d'eene deur geschildert
was Platoos Hol: daar elk door schaduw-liefd' verwildert;
An d'ander deur daar zachmen Kebes tafereel

APPENDIX 4

The epigram of the *Antrum Platonicum*.

Maxima pars hominum cecis immersa tenebris
Volvitur assidue, et studio letatur inani:
Adspice ut obiectis obtutus inhereat umbris,
Ut veri simulacra omnes mirentur amentque

Et stolidi vana ludantur imagine rerum.
Quam pauci meliore luto, qui in lumine puro
Secreti a stolida turba, ludibria cernunt
Rerum umbras rectaque expendunt omnia lance:

Hi posita erroris nebula dignoscere possunt
Vera bona, atque alios ceca sub nocte latentes
Extrahere in claram lucem conantur, at illis
Nullus amor lucis, tanta est rationis egestas.

APPENDIX 5

Hertspiegel 6. 492-497, Veenstra 168-169.

die meest doch blijven lijkewel in t'hert verkeert,
vol mis-verstant, vol zond, trots gulzich, en putierich,
vol Faam, staat, eer-gezoek, luij, toornich, nijdich, gierich:
Maar boven al goett-dunkend', en vol hovaardij,
klein achtens' alle menschen die niett zoo als zij
in hòòre-zeggens school zijn beu van boeck-waij-koeken

APPENDIX 6

Hertspiegel 6. 45-47, Veenstra 147.

T'is derthien laar geléen, datt ghij om te grondeeren
dit griexsche statt; griex leerd', nu kom ik 't u vol-leeren.
Ditt boek, en beeld-schrifts-puijk heeft veel verborghen zin;
T'is ijglijx levens beelt.

NOTES

I thank Lucy Schlüter who has patiently listened, read, criticized and contributed in the course of the writing of this work. I thank Kenneth Ellison Davis for his translation of my Dutch text. I also thank Carol and Alex Adler, Corrie Bakels, Jos Biemans, Sible de Blaauw, Herman Brijder, Claudine Chavannes, Harm-Jan van Dam, Trudy Dunning-Kattouw, Peter Engelfriet, Marijke Gumbert, Chris Heesakkers, Bram Kempers, Carla Maigret, Bert Meijer, Aafke van Oppenraay, Edwin Rabbie, Johan Schenk and Anton Zeven.

1   For the hearts by Leonardo, see Clark 3, 19029r, 19062, 19065r, 19071-19073, 19084r, 19087, 19126r.

2   Alcalde del Rio fig.57, Pl. 44. Following the original publication of this work, my attention was drawn to the article by Werner Nebel, which was published in 1935. I was surprised to note that its subject was the 'Panofsky problem': 'Das symbolische Kartenherz, wie es uns im täglichen Leben häufig, etwa als Schmuckgegenstand oder Warenzeichen, begegnet, hat, wie auch der Nichtmediziner weiß, nur noch eine sehr geringe Ähnlichkeit mit seinem ursprünglichen anatomischen Vorbild.' Was Panofsky aware of the article? Whilst it would seem highly likely that he was, the question must perforce remain unanswered. What is certain, however, is that Nebel also makes reference to the heart of the prehistoric elephant in the Pindal cave.

3   Lewinsohn 12-16.

4   The Olmec effigy vessel is in a private collection, Coe 251, Bendersky *passim*. The first two hearts of figure. 6 were published by Robicsek fig.4, the third by Rieff Anawalt 176.

5   Plutarch, *Isis and Osiris* 378, Babbitt 5. 159. The drawing of the heart urns in figure 7 are from Singer 1957, 7. The Egyptians wore heart amulets, prophylactic charms in the shape of a

funerary urn, Flinders Petrie 10, Pl. 1. Also Harris 89 and Brunner *passim*. Occasionally, the Egyptian heart urns bear remarkably little resemblance to a pitcher and remarkably more resemblance to an actual heart. For example, the one featured on the scales in the Book of the dead of Ani (British museum), dating from the fourteenth century B.C., as featured in Perry's article. However, contrary to what the writer says, this illustration does not appear to have been copied from Wallis Budge's publication, but rather from Dondelinger's book. In comparing the latter with the former, it is clear that what we have is a distorted representation of a conventional heart urn, the distortion having resulted from a certain unevenness in the papyrus.

The hearts of deceased European royalty and nobility were sometimes preserved separately in urns or vases down to the eighteenth century. See also Borgheer 36.

6   Aristotle, *History of animals* 1.17.496a, Peck 65.

7   *Hippocratic writings* 347-351. This short treatise on the heart may have been written by a near contemporary of Erasistratus of Ceos, a physician who was active about 260 BC. Others believe Philistus of Syracuse (fourth century BC) to be the author. For a discussion of authorship and dating of this text, see Harris 83 ff.

8   Galen, *On the usefulness of the parts of the body* 6.7, May 291, Harris 268.

9   Avicenna, *Canon* 3. 11. 1, Koning 686.

10   The passages from Avicenna, Rhazes and Hali Abbas were translated from Koning 686, 345 and 63.

11   Mesue 1. 34, Pagel 33. There is little specific information about Mesue. There was a Christian physician of this name who is thought to have come from the Near East in either the eleventh or twelfth century. He is believed to have studied in Baghdad and to have been strongly influenced by Avicenna. Works ascribed to him probably have been translated from Arabic

into Latin, Pagel 137, Pellegrino 15-23. Albertus Magnus 1. 3. 4. 577, Stadler 206. Mondeville 14a, 59: *cor habet formam pineatam*. Mundinus (Wickersheimer 33): *est figuras vel pyramidalis*. 'A work upon any science or art, as says Galen, is issued (...) that he may be saved from the oblivion of old age', Pilcher 322. This phrasing was frequently used by later writers. Singer (1955, 93) wrote about Mundinus: 'His personal influence and enthusiasm no doubt helped also towards the phenomenal success of his work, which for two hundred years held a position without rival as the text-book of the medical schools of Italy, where (according to Adelphus) even as late as the sixteenth century Mondino 'was still worshipped by all the students as a very god'.

12   Chauliac 56, *Fruehe Anatomie* 111.

13   In his *Fabrica* (1543, 6.8), Vesalius still calls the heart pine-cone-shaped and its base round. *Gray's anatomy* 1475, fig.10.28. Harris 85.

14   The religous interest in the association of love with the heart can be ascribed to the influence of the works, amongst others, of Saint Augustine, Boethius and Pope Gregory the Great. The Heart of Jesus, as the focus of his love for mankind and the source of the blood he shed for the redemption of the world, features in religious texts from the eleventh century onwards, including, for example, those of Saint Bernard, Charbonneau 99. It also started to become popular in religious art at the beginning of the thirteenth century, primarily through the writings of mystics like the German nuns Hildegard of Bingen, Mechteld of Magdeburg and Gertrude the Great, who were writing between 1150 and 1300, but equally because of the writings of, for example, SS Francis of Assisi, Bonaventura and Antony of Padua. For the Heart of Jesus, see also note 68. See also Bietenholz *passim*.

15   The Siana cup by the Taras painter is in the Allard Pierson museum in Amsterdam, Brijder figs. 12, 13. The Caere hydra is in the Villa Giulia, Rome, Schefold 145. The amphora is in the Staatliche Antiken Sammlung, Munich, Dietz 80. Erastes

and Eromenos on a dish by Douris, Martin von Wagner museum, Wuerzburg. The Roman inscriptions are taken from Rossi 3.19.7, 3.30.9 and 3.31.2, 80. The floor mosaic is in the Damas national museum, Balty 41. The lamp was found in Malta, Buhagiar 40. The Coptic textiles with red leaves is illustrated in Bourguet 1. D162. The second coptic textile, in the Vatican museum, is from the third century, Renner Pl. 29. The *pegasoi* are in the Musee historique des tissues, Lyons, Dietz 82. Lombardus' *Psalmen Kommentar* is in the State library, Bamberg. *Carmina burana* is in the Bavarian State library, Munich, Cem. 4660, f. 64v, Legner 484, Boeckler 61. The Omnipotent hand is above the crucifix in the apse of the San Clemente basilica, Rome. The antependium with the life of Mary is in the Augustinermuseum, Freiburg im Breisgau, Parler 1, Pl. 11. The Regensburg textile is in the town hall of Regensburg, Kurth 1. 231, 2. 110-112. The printer's mark is illustrated in Grimm 99. In the basilica of San Clemente, God's hand is shown clasping a few leafy figures held together by means of a string or tendril. In a miniature from the *Hortus deliciarum* (32), a twelfth-century Alsatian manuscript, He is similarly represented holding the Pentecostal tongues suspended by lines above the heads of the Apostles. The heart icon-shaped (ivy) leaf is frequently used as 'linear' border decoration, as well as in the form of elongated, tapering heart-icon-shaped leaves on Coptic textiles, and they are often red in colour. For heart-icon-shaped leaf ornaments on, for example, oil lamps from late Roman and Byzantine periods, see Buhagiar figs 11a, 20g, 118b, 368, 1b. See also the grey marble Asturian screen with heart-icon-shaped leaves, dating from the 9th century, in the church of San Miguel de Lino in Oviedo, Spain, *The art of Spain* fig.63b. Trees with heart-icon-shaped leaves frequently feature in medieval miniatures, e.g. Czech National library, cod. l. Germ. 92, 1r and 2r; Bavarian State library, Munich, cgm 6406, 131r. On heart-icon-shaped leaf ornaments see also Bietenholz *passim* and Jakobi 65 'lineares Ornament', 70 'Herzblatt', 71 'Pfeilblatt', 75 'Herzpalmettenfries'. Many of the ivy-shaped leaves are coloured red.

16   The fragment illustrated in figure 8 is in the Archeological institute of the University of Tuebingen, 18/3, Gladigow 352-353. There is a similar fragment in the Pergamon museum, Berlin, 30414, 110, Meer 56. The human heart measures 12 cm from base to tip, and is 8-9 cm in diameter, *Gray's anatomy* 1475.

17   Hermann 107, fig.4c, Forrer 1891, Pl. 16. Saints are not the only figures endowed with aureoles on Coptic textiles. They appear above the heads of various personalities, Greek gods, heroes or personifications of the seasons and even of ordinary mortals, such as that of a dancer, Bourget B20, B21, B25, C77, D42, F167-169, 174, 227, Wessel 1963 figs 110, 112, 113, 114, 132, Pl. 23, 214. A single-leaf motif in the background of a portrait, for example, is also to be found on a textile, Rutschowskaya 37 and Forrer 1893, Pl. 17.1. Three heart icon-shaped ornaments in green and yellow appear next to a figure with an aureole (Christ?) on a Coptic textile, illustrated in Forrer 1893, Pl. 17.6. There is a similar saintly figure, in this case with ornamental heart leaves with stalks and tendrils, in Forrer 1893, Pl. 17.3, see figure 99a.

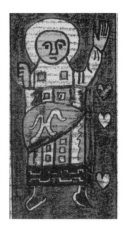 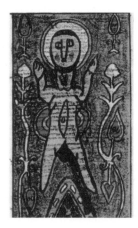

Fig. 99a. Figures with aureoles and heart icon-shaped ornaments on Coptic textiles, 4th century.

Ezekiel 36:26. I do not know of any representations of the prophet with a heart. The heart as an attribute of Saint Augustine is not found in art before the second half of the fourteenth century. See also note 39.

18 Aristotle's 'not elongated but roundish' in *History of animals* 1. 17, Peck 1965, 65. Galen, *On the usefulness of the parts of the body* 6. 7, May 291.

19 Macrobius, *Saturnalia* 1, 6, 17, 52.

20 *Hippocratic writings* 347, Harris 54. This text contains a description of a beating heart in a still living body. On opening the thorax, one can see the heart moving within the pericardium, which has a membranous, bladder-like shape. The Etruscan ex-voto with bladder-heart in Berlin was published by Sudhoff 1907, Pl. 22. The Roman bladder heart is part of a polyvisceral ex-voto in the Archeological museum, Florence, inv. no. 80757. For an outline of its organs, see figure 100, Singer 1957, 41.

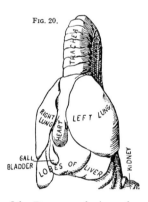

Fig.100. Outline of the Roman polyvisceral ex-voto in figure 11.

The ex-votos of separate hearts, to the right in figure 11 (Regnault fig.5), allow one to see them with the remnants of the excised blood vessels at the base. They recall to mind the frayed base of the Mesoamerican hearts (figure 6 on page 11). See also notes 30, 32, 36 and 91. The upper model in figure 11 is asymmetrical; here, the lesser half of the heart has been turned to the front. Regnault ascribes this asymmetry to the fact that, on death, the right chamber contracts more markedly, because its wall is thinner than that of the left chamber.

21 Leaves were also painted in red in the middle ages. The ornamental spade leaves on the *chlamys* of Saint Demetrius on an eleventh-century Byzantine enamel are red. Wessel 1967, 36. There is no connection between this saint and the heart, so here too we must take the pattern in the material of the robe to be a leaf motif. Some of the ivy-shaped leaves are coloured red in an early thirteenth-century herbarium, see *Medicina antiqua* 26r, 36r, 39r, 52v, 114r, 144v. The Dionysos (Bacchus) portrait in figure 12 is from the 5th century, Bourguet B20, Wessel 223, fig.110. For another Dionysos with nimbus, see Wessel fig.112. This, and the textile with the Spring, whose (female) personification is also represented with an aureole and a single attribute to the right of the head, is from the fifth century, Bourguet B25. It is surrounded by green and red leaves. The dancer with the large leaf ornament is from the sixth century, Bourguet C26. All these textiles are in the Louvre, Paris. Other heart-icon-shaped forms are the ornamental arrowheads, which are found in the Middle East, and in Coptic and medieval European art (Jansma *passim,* Depuydt *passim),* on a tenth-century Andalusian dish (*The art of medieval Spain* fig.52) and in the San Isidoro Bible, dated 960 (*ibid.* 122).

22 Plutarch, see note 5.

23 At the beginning of the third millennium B.C., the heart and the tongue were regarded in Egypt as the body's most important organs; the former as the seat of intelligence; the latter as the executor of the will of the heart, Brunner 9. One might also recall Isaiah 32:4: 'The heart also of the rash shall understand knowledge, and the tongue of the stammerers shall be ready to speak plainly'. In one of Perriere's emblems (1533, 73), the courtier, with his honeyed words, presents his tongue on a platter, thus symbolizing flattery, Henkel 1047. See also the heart-icon-shaped Pentecostal tongues in the Omnipotent hand in the basilica of San Clemente in Rome, figure 8 and note 15.

24 Hahn-Woernle *passim, Heinrich der Loewe und seine Zeit* A1. 32. Wolf 97. The court allegedly was that of Otto IV, King of Sicily.

25 For illustrations of medieval maps, see Kugler *passim*. As is the case with many other medieval world maps, the Ebstorf map is associated with the body of Christ, his head being drawn at the upper edge (the east), his hands on the left and right sides and his feet at the base. Jerusalem is placed in the middle, thus implying that its placement makes it the heart of the map. Sicily's placement in the map, projected on to the human body, would locate it on the upper left leg. This too makes its improbable that the outline of the island was intended to represent a heart.

26 In the first edition of this work (1999), it was stated at this point in the text that a barbarian in one of the details in the Ebstorf map, is eating a classical pyramid-shaped heart. Such is not the case; he is in fact consuming a foot sliced off from the victim by another barbarian.

27 The Andalusian heart box is illustrated in *The art of medieval Spain AD 400-1200*, 46. Although one cannot say with certainty, it is not unlikely that the shape of these boxes was meant to represent a heart. 'The heart shape (...) is unusual in the Islamic repertoire, and the absence of Arabic inscriptions points to the possibility that they were produced for the Christian community in the *taifa* period'. The Cambridge heart sketch is from manuscript 428/428, fol. 50, Gonville and Caius college, Cambridge, Singer 1922, 39, Singer 1957, 66. The combination of the words *heart*, *hot* and *dry* is regularly found in medieval texts, e.g. in the twelfth-century *Anatomia magistri Nicolai physici* and in the thirteenth-century *Anatomia vivorum*, Corner 75, 108. Chauliac 33: 'les medicus [i.e. the classical authors, philosophers] argruent le couer estre chaud et sec'. For the 'innate heat' of the heart, see also note 113. The black pointed protuberance from the heart base could also represent the remnant of a blood vessel, similar to the frayed heart base as described in notes 20, 30, 32, 36 and 91.

28 Figure 16 is taken from *Compendium medicinae*, a thirteenth-century manuscript in which the human internal organs are associated with the signs of the zodiac, Gurrieri 36. Such figures, often of a blood-letting man, occur until the sixteenth century. The

heart is always connected with the Leo sign of the zodiac. Figure 16, second illustration, is from the *Codex Trivulziano*, Belloni fig.2. The 'arrow' through the heart represents the arterial tree, Gurrieri 37. For the arterial tree, see also notes 30 and 66.

29 The Pruefening manuscript is in the Bavarian State library, Munich. See also *Regensburger Buchmalerei* 34. The illustration from *Glossarium Salomonis* was published by Sudhoff 1907, Pl. 13. See also Frank 50. The influence of the ancient and medieval methods of anatomical instruction with the use of a number of plates can still be traced in the sixteenth century, for example in the six plates that Vesalius used in his *Tabulae anatomiae sex* (1538).

30 The Caius heart is a separate heart sketch from manuscript 190/223 in Gonville and Caius college, Cambridge. The heart in the Pisa manuscript was referred to in the older literature as Codex Roncioni, Pisa University 735 (formerly Ronc. 99). It was published by Sudhoff 1914, Pl. 14. In medieval anatomical literature, the heart base was called 'radix' (i.e. root, of the vessels), Chauliac 1.2.5, Keil 37. The shoots emerging from the base remind one of the leafy stems and tendrils in the Roman catacombs (see figure 8 on page 17 and page 84). However, the shoots emerging from the base of the heart in figure 18 on page 29 could only be taken to signify the 'tree of vessels' or the 'arterial tree', see Galen: 'from the heart springs out an artery in the same manner as does the trunk of a tree from the earth (...) on the great artery, before it breaks up into two subdivisions, you can see two off-shoots like that which emerges from the seed of a plant when it germinates (...) the artery springing out from the heart divides itself just as the trunk of a tree divides into branches', Duckworth 172, 173. This metaphor was used, quite literally, by Perriere in an emblem in his *Morosophie* (1553, 97), Henkel 145, see figure 101. There are many variations of the arterial tree. For example, Baumgarten's printer's mark (the last picture in figure 8), and in a seal (figure 51). Mansur's five-picture series appeared in an illustrated Persian monograph on anatomy, the *Tashrih bi al-Tasurr*, which was compiled in 1396. There is a manuscript (46) in the Royal college of

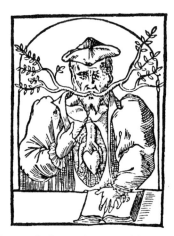

Fig.101. Guillaume de la Perriere's emblem with a heart tree.

physicians, London, Schott Pl. 1, fig.2, Sudhoff 1908, Pl. 15. Mondeville's heart sketch is from manuscript 227, fol. 226r. Royal college of physicians, London.

31   Hippocrates, *The heart* 7. 8, Lloyd 250, 349. Galen, *On anatomical procedures* 7. 8, 9, 11, 15, Singer 1956, 181, 184, 189, 196. Galen, *On the usefulness of the parts of the body* 6.15, May 316, Harris 273, 274. Avicenna, *Canon* 3. 11. 1, Koning 686. Albertus Magnus 1. 3. 4. 580, Stadler 207. The 'ears' of the heart were mentioned in most medieval anatomical works, including the twelfth-century *Anatomia magistri Nicolai physici*, Corner 76. For Estienne's heart, see Singer and Rabin 19, fig.9. For Avicenna's description, see the quotation on page 14.

32   The heart of the Circulation man from figure 21 is from the same Caius manuscript (fol. 2v.) as mentioned in note 30. The Raudnitz heart is from a five-picture series, published by Sudhoff 1910, Pl. 9. The third sketch is from a German manuscript 49, fol. 36, Wellcome institute for the history of medicine, London, Seebohm *passim* and Saxl *passim*. Two of these hearts have ears. See also the isolated heart sketch from the Caius manuscript in figure 18 on page 29.
For the black spot as a grain of seed, see Haneveld 265.
Galen situates the *os cordis* at the base, where the large vessels emerge (*On anatomical procedures* 7. 10. 618-622, Singer 1956,

186-188). The hard and strong fibrous tissue in the base of the heart was probably mistaken for bone or cartilage tissue. Although Aristotle also locates the *os cordis* in the base *(History of animals* 2.15. 506a, *Parts of animals* 3. 4. 666b, Harris 134), Galen was not in agreement with Aristotle on this point either *(On the usefulness of the parts of the body* 6. 19, May 326, Harris 280 and *On anatomical procedures* 7. 8, 10. 618-619, Singer 1956, 186). The polemical tone with which he describes the positive result of his research on the heart bone recalls the way he refutes the difference in size between the two chambers or the existence of the third ventricle as described by Aristotle.

The heart bone is regularly mentioned in medieval literature, for example by Avicenna, *Canon* 3, Koning 686, 690, Albertus Magnus 1, 3, 4, 577, Stadler 206, and Chauliac, Nicaise 56. The bone was still mentioned and, in a phantasized form, separately illustrated in more sophisticated anatomical plates of the skeletons around 1500, Sudhoff 1908, 46, 48, figs 2, 3. It was never pictured inside the heart, not even inside the body. It was not until the middle of the sixteenth century that the authority of Vesalius put an end to the hypothetical heart bone by declaring that it is not found in the human heart. The most likely explanation is that the black tip sticking out of the base in the Cambridge sketch of the heart (figure 15 on page 26) represents remains of excised vessels. See also notes 20, 27, 30, 36 and 91.

33   For the Raudnitz heart and its accompanying Latin text, see Sudhoff 1910. The black spot is also mentioned in the text of a five-picture series dated 1420 (ms. 5000 in the Wellcome institute for the history of medicine, London): 'nigro grano quod est intus in corde in quo spiritus habitat', Hill 1959, 18. Hill (1965, 71) reported that the *nigrum granum* performs the function of the middle ventricle in Avicenna's system: it is the point at which *spiritus* is pumped into the arterial blood. The black grain in the heart and the pneuma circle(s) around it are regularly found in plates of the arterial and venous systems in the five-picture series. In the Raudnitz heart sketch in figure 22, there is a horizontal band which has been left open, so as to make it possible to see the *granum nigrum*, as well as the emerging blood vessels, in the centre. For the relevant Hippocratic passages on pneuma, see Deichgraeber 7, 9, 41;

for those by Aristotle, see Tricot 166, Frantzius 143, Balme 157; for Galen, see Singer 1956, 184, 251 note 152; for Mundinus, see Wickersheimer 34 and Lonie *passim*.

34   For the 'innate heat' of the heart, see also notes 27 and 113. The pneuma circles can be seen in one of the two circulation men in most of the five-picture series, for example, in the circulation man to the left in figure 17 on page 28. The concentric pneuma circles are also mentioned by Johannes Mesue, about 1100: 'cum a puncto [cordis] per crescentes circulos gradatim perveniat ad ultimam perfectionem', Pagel 33.

35   Hippocrates, *The heart* 4, Lloyd, 348. The first and second pictures of figure 23 are from the Oxford Bodleian Ashmolean manuscript 399, Sudhoff 1914 Pl. 15.4, Singer 1955, 88 fig.6. and Singer 1957, 74, fig.34. The third is from manuscript W.308 in the Stadtarchiv, Cologne, Sudhoff 1914, 378, fig.16. The fourth (Chinese) sketch is from Wang Honghan's *Yixue yanshi*, 1692, 307. A possible alternative interpretation of the small skirt around the base of this heart is that it represents the rolled-up pericardium, of which Galen wrote that it surrounds the base of the heart like a crown, *On anatomical procedures*, 7. 3, Singer 1956, 175. The Oxford manuscript 399, fol. 34 contains another hazelnut heart, one of the organs 'strewn around', in a miniature of what is the earliest known representation of a dissection, about 1290, Singer 1957, 74, see figure 102. The heart is located there next to the left lower leg of the operator.

Images dating from the eighteenth- or nineteenth centuries from a Tibetan monastery, now in the Museum fuer Volkenkunde und Vorgeschichte, Hamburg, show human hearts being offered up. They are still conical in shape and somewhat resemble the medieval European hazelnut hearts, Thomae 13, 37. Apparently, the scalloped heart icon had not yet then permeated through to Asiatic art. See also note 90.

36   The *Roman de la poire* manuscript is located at the Bibiothèque nationale in Paris (ms. fr. 2186) and was published under the title *Le roman de la poire par Tibaut* by Christiane Marchello-Nizia

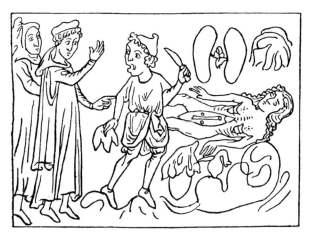

Fig. 102. Hazelnut heart, about 1290.

(Paris, 1984). The text quoted appears on folio 41 v, see Marchello-Nizia 62. The text within the letter 'S' reads: 'devant li se mist a genouz, le cuer que il tint en sa main, li mist si doucement el sain'; and the text within the letter 'M' reads: 'Ma dame a droit, qui m'envoie, son cuer a garder'. The initial 'S' appears on Plate 12 and the initial 'M' on Plate 16. (Lucy Schlüter brought this manuscript to my attention following the publication of the first edition of this work). See also Michael Camille, *The medieval art of love*, London, 1998, 29, from which certain sentences have been quoted here. For Giotto's *Caritas* see e.g. Previtali 354-355, fig.399-401. A small stalk appears to protrude from the base of this pine-cone heart. It probably represents an 'artery' (vessel or windpipe) emerging from the base of the heart. See also notes 20, 27, 30, 32 and 91. For the Aztec heart sacrifice, see Hagen 201. There is, of course, no historical connection with the depictions from Northern Italy.

37   Freyhan *passim*. Millard Meiss has attributed the panel, which was in a private collection, to the Master of the Stephaneschi altar. He considered it a unique representation: 'nowhere else is the Caritas group merged with the Madonna', Meiss 1978, 114-115, fig.169. The Saints and Virtues standing around the throne of the Madonna in the panel described by Meiss also appear on the mural in the Sala di Michelangelo of the Bargello museum, Florence (see figure 25 on page 35), but are so heavily damaged as to be almost unrecognizable.

38 We already find a twelfth-century picture of Caritas with a chalice on a capital of the Saint Lazare's church in Autun. Figure 27 on page 36 is a detail from a fresco from the lower church of San Francesco in Assisi. It shows Saint Francis being led by Jesus Christ to his bride, Poverty. In a recent study, the frescoes on these vaults are ascribed to Giotto, who is said to have designed them in 1322/1323 as a polemical stand in a difference of opinion between the Franciscan order and Pope John XXII about the monastic ruling in regard to poverty, Poeschke 47-48.

39 Gaddi's *Caritas* with a flame in the hand is on the second vault of the Baroncelli chapel of the Santa Croce, Florence, Ladis 105. See also note 42. Panofsky (39) and Freyhan (*passim*) provide sources from Hellenistic and Roman literature for the flame as an attribute of both Amor and Caritas. Also Luke 24:32: 'Did not our heart burn within us, while he talked with us by the way'. Fire or flame in the contamination of passion, love and heart is already suggested in The Song of Solomon (8:7); 'many waters cannot quench love, neither can the floods drown it'. The theme also occurs in an epigram by Callimachus (in the *Greek Anthology*, Paton 6): 'he is flaming with homoerotic fire' (Bing 135) or 'his flame is a man' (Mair 27). The torch of Amor dates back to Roman times; the heart burns with love in the work of Ovid, e.g. *Ars amatoria* 1. 80, and *Amores* 1, 1, 26. It occurs incidentally in twelfth-century courtly poetry, Ertzdorff 157b, 5: 'E'l feux, qu'il mou', and, more frequently, in *Carmina burana*, also from the twelfth century. 'Throughout the middle ages (...) probably influenced by the association of Amor and fire, Caritas itself was often compared to fire, light and flame', e.g. in Dante's *Purgatorio* (Freyhan 73-79).
In Dante's *Vita nuova*, Love forces the lady to eat of the lover's burning heart, Musa 120. The flaming heart features in the work, much admired by Dante, of Guido Guinizelli (1230-1276), one of the fathers of the dolce stil nuovo, Edwards 3.1, 4.2 and *passim*. The heart flaming from profane love is a common metaphor in Petrarch's poetry. The flaming heart as an attribute of Caritas makes its first appearance in Italian sculpture at the beginning of the fourteenth century. More than one Caritas with a flaming pine-cone heart was made by

Giovanni di Balduccio. An interesting one is the marble relief from about 1330, in the Samuel H. Kress collection in the National gallery of art, Washington, Middeldorf 7, fig.3, Freyhan Pl. 16d, see figure 103. With this Caritas figure, a

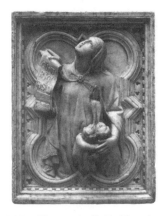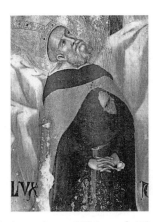

Fig.103. Giovanni di Balduccio, *Caritas*, about 1330, and Nicoletto Semitecolo, *Saint Augustine*, about 1360.

heart with a flame pointing upwards emerges from a tear in her garment, over the edge of which also flows a small waterfall of milk into the mouths of two children. In an earlier (1321) statue of Caritas by Tino da Camaino, two children suck from her breasts which are protruding through tears in her robe, Freyhan fig.16a. Somewhat later, on the base of a crucifix by Nicoletto Semitecolo in the Eremitani church in Padua, the heart of Saint Augustine protrudes in a similar way through a tear in his robe, Pallucchini fig.379, see figure 103.

In the *studiolo* in the Palazzo ducale in Urbino, there is a later Caritas (circa 1475) holding a large flaming object (a heart or a vessel), Cheles fig.61. The image of the heart for the love of God occurs frequently in religious literature from the thirteenth century onwards, also as the Heart of Jesus in which 'burns the great flame of love'.

40 Lorenzetti's first Caritas is now in the Palazzo municipale in Massa Marittima, see figure 104. Freyhan (81 and fig.15c) pointed to the similarity with the figure of Amor. An adult, crowned and winged Amor with outstretched arms, holding a

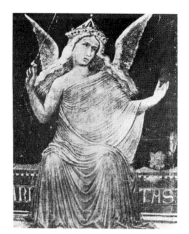
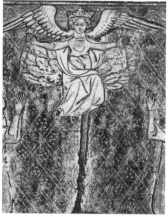

Fig.104. Ambrogio Lorenzetti's *Caritas,* 14th century, and *Amor* from a *Roman de la rose* manuscript, 13th century.

long arrow in each hand, had already featured in an early manuscript of the *Roman de la rose* (thirteenth century), Koenig 54. A similar Amor, but with a single long arrow in one hand and a flaming torch in the other, is shown in a fourteenth-century manuscript in the Bibliotheque nationale in Paris (1584 fol. 1v.), Panofsky fig.75, see figure 105. (A similar Amor

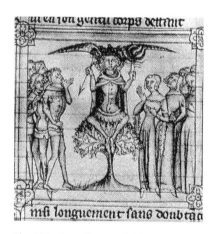
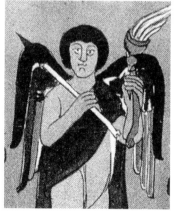

Fig.105. *Amor* from a 14th-century manuscript, and *Amor* from an 11th-century manuscript.

appears as late as 1490 in a woodcut of the *Ars memorativa* by Anton Sorg, Schramm, Pl. 364, 2952). Of a much earlier date is the adult winged Amor in an eleventh-century manuscript

146

of *De universo* by Hrabanus Maurus in Montecassino, which features him with a long arrow and flaming torch, Panofsky fig.71. Giotto and Dante referred to Caritas as 'amor'. As has been pointed out by Panofsky, Barberino's Amor was also an allegorical form, to which both religious and secular concepts had contributed, Freyhan 77. For Pisano's Caritas, see Venturi 2, 55, Pl. 10, 11. A Caritas caryatid with flaming pitcher, also by Giovanni Pisano, forms part of the pulpit of the Cathedral in Pisa, 1302-1311, Ayrton 157, 206, 226, fig.320. Another example is Andrea Guardi's Caritas with a flaming chalice on the chancel relief in the Maria della Spina church in Pisa, 1425, Kirschbaum 1. 350-351.

41   Bonaiuto's *Caritas* is in the Spanish chapel of Santa Maria Novella, Florence. Romano 191: 'Essa è reppresentata con due fiamma nelle mani e un 'altra sulla testa'. Bonaiuto's second Caritas in fig.35, was published by Marle 2. fig.28. Around 1460, in Francesco Pesellino's studio, a Caritas was painted with a flame on her right hand (and a child in her left arm), as one of the seven virtues, on a Florentine panel now in the Birmingham museum of art, Birmingham, Alabama, Shapley fig.303, see figure 106.

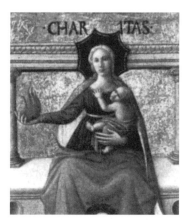

Fig.106. Francesco Pesellino and studio, *Caritas*, about 1460.

A closely similar figure with a flame in the hand was painted somewhat later in the studio of Piero Pollaiolo, Marle 2, fig.47. This Caritas in the Uffizi in Florence is also holding a flame directly between the fingers of her right hand, Marle 2. fig.36, Ettlinger Pl. 30. Caritas was not alone in being featured holding a flame in her hand. In a fourteenth-century French manuscript of the *Roman de la rose*, Venus is shown in a similar pose, with the flame also being a symbol of love, Kuhn Pl. 7, see figure 107.

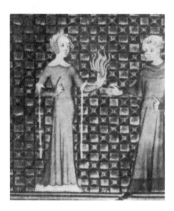

Fig.107. *Venus*, holding a flame in her hand, miniature from the *Roman de la rose*, 13th century.

From 1400 onwards, Saint Catherine of Siena was regularly depicted with a heart as attribute. She was also shown with either a flaming heart or a flame in the hand, albeit the distinction between the two is sometimes (no longer) clearly apparent. Relevant examples can be found in Kaftal 1952 and 1985, Kleinschmidt *passim*, and Bianchi *passim*. Although he too had a heart as attribute, Saint Antony of Padua is depicted more frequently holding a flame. An early example is Agnolo Gaddi's painting (1394) in the Santa Croce in Florence, Kleinschmidt 92. In Giovanni dal Ponte's triptych (1435), in the Vatican, he holds in his right hand a relatively big flame almost the size of an overlarge heart, Kaftal 1952, 86, 25e, fig.85. For other examples, see Kaftal 1968, 32k, fig.26, and Kleinschmidt *passim*. But Sassetta's early fifteenth-century Antony shows him holding a flaming heart, Kaftal 1952, 78, fig.73. And it is Antony of Padua and not, as previously identified, Bernardus, who stands in the background holding a flaming heart in Matteo di Giovanni's *Madonna with the Saints Nicolas and Bernardus* (Mayer 264).

I am aware of only one instance of Saint Catherine of Siena with a flaming heart as attribute (see figure 108). Since she is

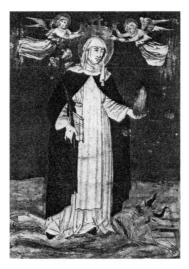

Fig.108. *Saint Catherine of Siena*, 14th century.

holding the tip of the heart upwards, the panel must be dated to the first half of the fourteenth century.

One of the vault frescoes in the Strozzi chapel in Santa Maria Novella, Florence, pictures Saint Thomas Aquinas as Love, holding a flaming heart with its tip pointing upwards. Kaftal (1952, 988, fig.1111) dates it '14th-15th century', but given the direction of the tip, a fourteenth-century dating is probably more precise.

42 Gaddi's overlarge (flaming) heart is on the south wall of the Baroncelli chapel of the Santa Croce, Florence. Ladis 107. Orcagna's Caritas is illustrated in Kreytenberg Pl. 61-64, the Caritas of Balduccio's in a close-up in Pope-Hennessy 1972, 26, 198-199, Pl. 61. For Rene of Anjou's manuscripts *Le mortifiement de vaine plaisance*, see Lyna, and *Le livre du cuer d'amour espris*, see Trenkler. Another large heart (with the flaming point still held upwards) can be seen in a fourteenth-century ivory originating from the Pisa school, Didron 57, see figure 109.
Wickersheimer 32. Mundinus derived this notion from Aristotle, who divided hearts by size into three different

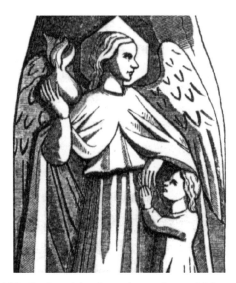

Fig.109. *Caritas* with a large heart, ivory, 14th century.

categories and claimed that the human heart belonged to the category of the largest. Aristotle, *History of animals* 3. 3. 513a, Peck 175 and *Parts of animals* 111. 4. 666b, Peck 243. Galen mentions 'the broad circular base above', *On the usefulness of the parts* 6. 7, May 291. Avicenna also calls the heart large (Koning 686). According to Hieronymo Manfredi's *Anatomy* (1490), the human heart size, compared with that of other animals, 'is very large' (Singer 1955, 122, 126). Augustine, *De unitate ecclesiae* 1.66. In a painting by Fra Angelico, dating from circa 1430, Saint Catherine of Siena is pictured with an overlarge, unscalloped heart next to the *Madonna del bambino* in the Santa Maria Novella in Florence, Bianchi 184, Pl. 16.1. See also Bianchi 183.There is a book illustration dating from the same period showing Saint Catherine with an large heart, Bianchi 85, see figure 110. And perhaps for the first time in his iconography, Saint Antony is shown holding a large, conical-shaped heart in a painting by Fiorenzo di Lorenzo, Kleinschmidt fig.56. The same is true for a depiction of Saint Augustine on a white linen embroidered sixteenth-century German altar-cloth in the Metropolitan museum of art, New York, 29. 87, see figure 110. Both are holding the heart by the tip.

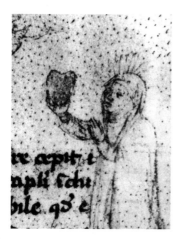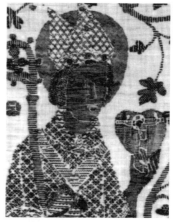

Fig.110. *Saint Catherine* with a large heart, first half of 15th century, and *Saint Augustine* with a large heart, German altar-cloth, 16th century.

43   Panofsky 115, note 64 and fig.88.

44   The mirror-case is in the Victoria and Albert museum, London, 217-1867, Barnet 227. A similar depiction is shown on a writing tablet, Barnet 237. The typical gesture of 'offering up' is also to be found on other amorous ivories from the same period, Koechlin 1109.

45   One of the last saints to be shown holding a heart aloft by its tip is Saint Antony on a panel by Sasetta, from the first half of the fifteenth century, Kaftal 1952, 25g. The Giovanni del Biondo panel is in the Vatican Pinacoteca, 40014, Mancinelli 113.
That Caritas and other virtues were sometimes pictured with a nimbus is clear from another Florentine panel in the Pinacoteca Vaticana, showing the *Madonna del parto with the personifications of the virtues* (1375-1380). The Caritas figure is represented there with a flaming cornucopia and a flaming heart which is also held by the tip, Mancinelli 111-113. There is a 'late' Caritas with a burning heart held by the tip in Netherlandish art in an engraving by J. Wierix entitled *The good death* from about 1550, Wierix 1494. From approximately the same period, we have the Caritas in an etching made by Dirck Coornhert after Maarten van Heemskerk, entitled *Knowledge of God bringing forth Charity*, Veldman 1990, 192 (see

figure 111) and the Caritas in a drawing by Pieter Bruegel, Muenz, Pl. 140.

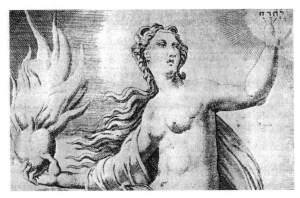

Fig.111. Dirck Coornhert, *Knowledge of God bringing forth Charity*, 1550.

A chapel of Notre Dame du Bourg in Rabastens, dedicated to Saint Augustine, contains a large mural on which an angel presents Sigisbert with Augustine's flaming heart. This heart is scalloped, it is held by the tip and it is burning from the base, Courcelle 46. 7, Pl. 45. This is inconsistent, iconographically, with the painting's early fourteenth-century provenance. The explanation may be that, shortly after 1860, the murals were painted over and it would seem that, on that occasion, a fifteenth-century (or later) heart shape was introduced.

46   For Barberino's *Documenti d'amore* see Panofsky 117-120, note 68, fig.90 and Egidi (1902) *passim*, figure facing page 8 and Partsch 79-87, Pl. 48. If we assume that Balduccio's heart is scalloped, we must perforce accept a number of very unusual aspects of it: the base is not uppermost, the tip inclines to the right side of the body and the flame is not emerging form the base, but from the side of the right chamber. The German tapestry is in Regensburg. The winged heart appears already in one of Petrarch's sonnets as 'cori impenna' (Durling 177 and, by implication, in 139 and 335). The image occurs more frequently in the latter part of the fifteenth century, particularly in the miniatures of the *Livre de cuer d'amours espris* by Rene of Anjou, Trenkler *passim,* and Koenig *passim.* The winged heart became a more common theme in later

Petrarchist poetry and in emblematics, Yates 118, 120 and *passim*. The French tapestries of figure 40 are in the Louvre in Paris. An early example of a scalloped heart (1406-1408) in art is the representation of *Venus and her children* in Christine de Pisan's manuscript *Epitre d'Othea*, Bibliotheque nationale, Paris 606, 6r, Parler 3.86, Meiss 1974, 2. 87, see figure 112.

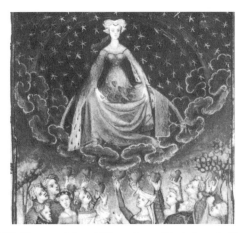

Fig.112. *Venus and her children*, from Christine de Pisan's
Epitre d'Othea, circa 1407.

47   Janssen 31, Bachmann *passim*.

48   The illustration is from the fourteenth-century manuscript no. 1187 of the *Gran conquista de ultramar*, manuscript 1187, Biblioteca nacional, Madrid. Jean de Vingle's mark, is from Davies 105. In this device, the heart icon has the same shape as that used for depicting an heraldic shield. For figure 42, see Davies 149, 179, 177. An earlier version of Rugerius' device, dated 1488, is one of the first Italian instances of the transformation of the orb into the shield shape, Davies 179. For the development of the heart icon from the orb, see Davies 177: 'This [i.e. Levet's] may be the earliest heart-shape to appear anywhere in a printers' mark, the earliest in Italy being Stagnino's 1493 (...). This outline shape may have originated in Italy from the orb (which it evidently represents), the first suggestion of it being the slight point added to the base [of an orb] as seen in Pasquale's, this soon being developed into a

distinct V-form and shortly afterwards into the heater shield so often seen in Italy and at Lyons. Thus, it seems that all these [heart] shapes and later aberrations are derived from the orb or globe in the first place.'

The heart surmounted by a cross came to assume the meaning of the Heart of Jesus in the second half of the fourteenth century, though it bore this meaning much earlier in literature. Round about 1500, we find printers' marks featuring the orb as well as the heart surmounted by a cross, e.g. in the devices of Gorge Costilla and Petrus Jacobi, Davies 186, 46.

49 Wickersheimer Pl. 2, fig.8. Vigevano provides a more realistic representation than his predecessors of the relative size of the heart and of the lungs.

50 For the double apex, see Galen, *On anatomical procedures* 7. 11. 623, Singer 1956, 188, note 159, Harris 274.

51 For the texts of Aristotle, Hippocrates, Plato and Galen, see May 18, 20, 620-621. For Galen, see also Goss 1962, 80. Albertus Magnus: 'Matrices autem in omnibus habent divisionem in duo', Stadler 995. For Gratheus, see Birkhan 78, miniature 17. Berengario 78-81. Chauliac (1363) : 'L' amarry [uterus]... n'ait que deux seins, ou cavitez manifestes', Nicaise 67.

52 Albertus Magnus 1.3.4.577 on the heart: 'ventribus basis eius (...) indivisio'.

53 The passages on the medical school of Bologna and its scholars are derived from Singer 1957 and Singer 1962. For the passage from Aristotle, see also Harris 123, 125, 135 and Peck 1. 175.

54 Galen denied the existence of a third ventricle: 'At the point where this is to be located, according to Aristotle, there is a dilation (*fovea*) of the right ventricle at the base of the heart; no third ventricle', *De venarum arteriarumque dissectione* 9, *On the usefulness of the parts of the body*, 6.9, May 295, *On anatomical proceedures*, 13. 5. 195, *Duckworth* 156. It is assumed by some

authors that Galen's 'cavity in the right chamber' was a reference to the *conus arteriosus*, from which the pulmonary vessels emerge, Goss 1961, 364, May 245. See also figure 45 on page 52.

55 Avicenna, *Canon* 3.11.1. This passage from the *editio princeps* of Cremona's Latin translation of Avicenna (fol. 96r) runs as follows: 'Et in ipso sunt tres ventres, scilicet duo ventres magni et venter quasi medius quem Galienus nominavit foveam aut meatum non ventrem, ut sit ei receptaculum (...) Et inter ambos sunt viae ut meatus'. This quotation, and the introductory sentence to it, are from Singer 1955, 128.

56 Alfredus Anglicus 4 and 5, Baeumker 14-19. For Ricardus, see Corner 108.

57 Albertus Magnus 1. 3. 4, Stadler 578. Bartholomew Anglicus' text is quoted by Singer 1955, 129.

58 In 1304 Mondeville gave lectures and demonstrations in anatomy for students in Montpellier. He followed the conventional practice by using plates. The originals have long since been lost, but they must have resembled the miniatures with full-length figures that appeared in the French translation of Mondeville's latin book of anatomy first written in 1314, MacKinney 237. In addition, he certainly used plates on which the individual organs were outlined, various versions of which were in circulation. The organ sketches in figures 18 on page 29, 21 on page 31, 22, 46 on page 54 and 47 are from didactic plates of this kind. Numerous copies and notes of Mondeville's and his colleagues' anatomical lessons went the rounds. Anatomical sketches were sometimes made as marginal annotations in manuscripts or lecture notes, see, for example, the second diagram in figure 18 on page 29 and those in figure 46. The first pen drawing of the heart in figure 46 is from a Mondeville manuscript in Erfurt, published by Sudhoff 1908, 88, Pl. 24. 10. The second is from a manuscript in the Staatsbibliothek, Berlin (lat. fol. 219, 84v). The relevant French text of Mondeville runs as follows: 'Le cuer a .2. ventrauz, c'est .2. concavités; la concavite senestre est plus

haute que la destre pour l'asise du cuer qui est ainsi. Ou milieu de ces .2. concavites est une parai moienne, en la quele parai ou milieu de la partie desous est une concavite qui est apelee le .3. ventrail d'aucuns', Bos 91, 315-316. The anatomy book by Mundinus (1316) contains the same description as that of Mondeville; in that part of his text where he starts to cut the heart open from the apex, one could even read that he also considered the third ventricle to be situated close to the tip of the heart, as is the case in Mondeville's sketches, Wickersheimer 33, 34. For Avicenna's quotation, see page 100 and note 111.

59 Mesue 1, 34, Pagel 1893, 33. That Mesue assumed a vertical arrangement of the chambers of the heart may have resulted from a misunderstanding of ancient or medieval texts, which indicated that one of the two chambers progressed further downwards than the other and, as a result, occcupied the major part of the tip of the heart. That medieval writers sometimes did not even visualise what they read or copied is clear from the fact that in a later passage Mesue refers simply to the two chambers of the heart, the right and the left.

60 For the confusion occurring in accounts of the heart as a result of Aristotle's postulate of the third ventricle, see Harris *passim*, Lambert 391. The Mundinus passages are from Wickersheimer's edition (34) of the first printed version (1478) of the *Anathomia* (1316). Chauliac 1976, 37. For the Middle English version of Chauliac's *Anatomy*, see Wallner 1964, 112 and Wallner 1995, 50.

61 It is remarkable that two early sketches of the heart more faithfully reflect the classical texts than most fourteenth-century images. The Cambridge heart from circa 1100 (figure 15 on page 26) shows the third ventricle centred in the base of the heart. The thirteenth-century Pisa heart (figure 18 on page 29) also shows the third ventricle at the centre of the heart, as it were 'in the thickness of the septum', as Mundinus was to write a century later.

62 Chauliac 1.6, Wallner 1964, 128: 'the galle is a purse or a

pannicler vesic, sette in the concauitee of the lyuer about the myddes penule or lobe'.

63 Aristotle, *History of animals* 3. 3. 513b, Peck 175: 'Thus the blood-vessel passes through the heart'. For the quotation from Avicenna see Koning 687 and Singer 1995, 127. Even Vesalius, who cannot have seen the openings in the septum between the two chambers of the heart, would seem to have assumed, without sound evidence, that blood must flow from the right to the left side of the heart.

64 The heart from the Raudnitz Circulation man in figure 48 on page 59 is from Sudhoff 1910, 356, Pl. 8, 9 (see also figure 21 on page 31); those from Hundt and Peyligk were published by Herrlinger figs 91 and 94.

65 Hippocrates described the external division between the right and left halves of the heart as a 'stitch' ('the right ventricle appearing (...) as if it had been sewn on from the outside', *Hippocratic writings, The heart* 4, Harris 86). Aristotle referred to it as 'a sort of articulation, which resembles the sutures of the skull', Aristotle, *Parts of animals* 3. 4, Peck 243. Galen pointed out the difference in substance of the walls of the chambers; the left side is thick and hard, while 'the right side is thin and soft, and it often has an outline of its own', Galen, *On anatomical procedures* 7. 11. 625, Singer 1956, 188; *On the usefulness of the parts of the body* 6. 16, May 319. The diagram of the heart in the Cambridge manuscript (figure 15 on page 26) also features a vertical line, but since this sketch is a cross-section, it represents the septum and not the sulcus. If Peyligk's heart (figure 49 on page 60) is not a cross-section but a frontal view, then the vertical furrow in the latter is intended to stand for the *sulcus* and not for the third chamber. The dip and the sulcus appear, incorrectly, to be clearly indicated on the sketch of the heart of one of the pregnant women in the anatomy book of the fifteenth-century Viennese professor Johannes de Ketham (see figure 113), whose illustrations go back to late medieval prototypes. But this is not the case; in fact, in this sketch the conical lung partially overlaps the left side of the conical heart. For Ketham, see also note 73 and

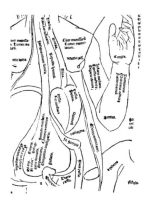

Fig.113. Johannes de Ketham, *Tabula tertia de muliere*, 15th century.

figure 116 on page 162. For Vesalius' heart, see Saunders Pl. 64.1.

66   For the seal of Esteme Couret, see Charbonneau-Lassay, 99. For the arterial tree in watermarks, see Briquet 3, and *passim*. See also note 30. The heart icon with a cross on the base started to appear in water- and printers' marks from the early 1400s, Briquet 3, 4310 and *passim*. Later on, we also see a cross (with a bunch of lilies) sticking out of the heart base, in the hand of a marble sculpture of Saint Catherine by Pietro Bernini from (1603-1606), in the church of the Girolamini or San Filippo Neri, Ruffo chapel, Naples, Bianchi 489, also 204, 363, 369, 378, 387, 391, 403, 404. For the Heart of Jesus, see also note 68.

67   Lewinsohn 85, fig.16, 17. For the sketches of figure 53, see Briquet 2. 4178, 4179, 4182, 4183, 4228, 4230, 4188, 4238, 4241, 4257. For a survey of the numerous watermarks with leaf decorations (spade leaves or clover) down to modern times, see Piccard *passim*.

68   The watermarks often comprised imposing attributes, such as the 'royal star' and the 'royal crown', because the customers of the paper factories were important individuals and bodies. The marks in figure 54 are from Briquet 3. 4291, 4328 and 4329. For watermarks with crowned heart, see Briquet 3. 4313-4330, with a star in Briquet 3. 4240-4253. A crowned

heart also appears in sixteenth-century printers' marks, for example, Matthias Jacob of Cologne, Grimm 312. See also note 48. Galen described the two coronary arteries as a wreath (*peristefanosa*), encircling, enwreathing or crowning the broad section of the heart, Galen, *On anatomical procedures* 7. 10, Singer 1956, 186, 618, also 13. 9. 216 and *On the usefulness of the parts of the body* 6, 14, 17, 18, May 325, 326. Harris (277) translated the latter passage about these vessels as forming 'a crown around the heart, for they call it the coronary'. See also Kuehn 3, 476.

The image of the crowned heart, as was later to appear in water- and printers' marks, perhaps refers to the metaphor of the heart of the king, which frequently occurs in the Bible e.g. in Proverbs 21:1 ('The King's heart is in the hand of the Lord', beautifully illustrated as a crowned heart in Montenay's emblem 30), also Proverbs 25:3, 2 Samuel 14:1, 2, Ezra 6:22, Jeremiah 4:9, Daniel 11:27. The later image of the Crown of thorns encircling the Heart of Jesus is perhaps linked to these texts. See also note 14. A late image of the Heart of Christ, surrounded by all the relevant attributes, is featured on a devotional picture from the Sacre Coeur in Paris. Dating from the first quarter of this century, it shows a flame issuing from the entrance of the red heart. Placed in the entrance is a halo-ed cross. The heart is bleeding from a wound. Both the

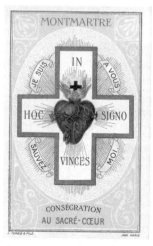

Fig.114. Devotional picture from the Sacre Coeur, Paris.

coronary heart vessels and a Crown of thorns encircle the broad section of the heart, see figure114. For Galen on the pericardium, see note 35.

69   The cloven heart in figure 54 is from an encyclopaedic manuscript (49, fol. 59r) of German origin, in the Wellcome institute for the history of medicine, London: 'Narrat valerius in speculo historiali Quod pietas vel compassio depingebatur sic in similitudinem hominis habentis in manu sua cor scissum in duas partes (...) Ad propositum Tota pictura patet spiritualiter de corde scisso in signum quod deus habuit cor scissum propter amorem nostrum et liberacionem Ita quilibet homo debet habere cor scissum Omni iuste petenti et maxime pauperibus et degentibus'. Valerius is incorrectly identified in the beginning of this quotation; the real author's identity is unknown. A similar Pietas (see figure 115) appears in an early fifteenth-century German manuscript in the Biblioteca

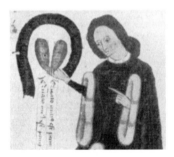

Fig.115. *Pietas* with cloven heart, early 15th century

Casanatense in Rome, Saxl 1927, 118, 11v, and Liebeschuetz 53 and Pl. 14: 'pietas vel compassio depingebatur in similitudine hominis habentis in manu sua cor scissum in duas partes'. See also Saxl 1942 *passim*. Guinizelli: 'che' per mezzo lo cor me lanciò un dardo, ched oltre 'n parte lo taglia e divide', Edwards 32. For Guinizelli, see also note 39. The dead miser's heart appears on the altar-piece by Hans Fries in the Franciscan church in Freiburg im Breisgau. Furmerius 13. For the engraving by Dirck Coornhert, *Penitent man brings forth the Truth*, see Veldman 1990, 91, fig.33, where reference is made to a second cloven heart engraved by Dirck Coornhert. On the right of the *Tabula Cebetis* by Hendrick Goltzius (figure 93 on page 113) there stands a female figure, Penitudo, with a cloven heart in her hand. A deeply cloven heart bearing the text 'fac bona, fuge malum' is an attribute in the hand of *The natural or pagan law* in an engraving by Baltens after Maarten de Vos, illustrated in Wierix fig.13.

70 Psalms 69:20, 147:3. Also: Psalms 34:19, 51:19, Isaiah 61:1, Numbers 32:9. (*Vulgata:* Psalms 68:21, 146:3, 33:19, 50:19). Reason was one of the symbolical figures present during Duke Matthew's triumphal entry into Brussels on 18 January 1578, Houwaert 24.

71 Aristotle, *Parts of animals* 3. 3. 665a, Peck 233: 'the windpipe which lead[s] to the lung and the heart'. Galen, *On the usefulness of the parts of the body* 7. 3. 'From late antiquity until the seventeenth century, most discussions of the heart and lungs by Byzantine, Arabic and European writers were largely based, directly or indirectly, on Galen's *De usum partium.* (...) The preparation of these accounts generally involved considerable selection and condensation of Galen's rather lengthy arguments, and in particular his long and nuanced discussion of the two pulmonary vessels was commonly reduced to a few aphoristic statements' (Bylebyl 218).

72 Galen, *On the usefulness of the parts of the body* 6.16, 7.2.3.6, 13.6, May 242, note 101, 321, 336, 337, 344-349, 602. The incorrect assumption about the respiration continued to exist in the middle ages. Writing in about 1210, Alfredus Anglicus said that the windpipe branched out into the lungs and finally ended up in the left chamber of the heart. 'Tracheae enim inferior extremitas multas et parvas venas quasi corporis sui radices per totam pulmonis substantiam dispergit, quarum una sinistrum cordis thalamum', Baeumker 15, 5-15.

73 Albertus 'trachea vero sive canna' is from *De animalibus* 13. 4, Stadler 894. The thirteenth-century trachea heart in figure 56 on page 68 is from the circulation man of the five-picture series of the Caius manuscript 190/223, see note 30. Donatello's relief is in the basilica of Saint Antony in Padua, Pope-Hennessy 1993,

223-224. The Gersdorff illustration is from his *Feldt und Stattbuch bewerter Wundartznei*, Frankfurt 1556, Singer 1955, 129. The woodcut had appeared before in Berengario's *Isagogae breves* in 1523. Here, 'the vessel' which Gersdorff (incorrecty) called the trachea, was correctly identified as the aorta, the name of which was part of the woodcut. Obviously, both pictures were copied from an earlier one. The Wound man's trachea heart is from Hieronymus Brunschwig, *Dis is das Buch der Cirurgia*, Strasbourg about 1485, Sudhoff 1907, 83, fig.32. The two Chinese drawings are from *Tabulae anatomicae* in the Staatsbibliothek, Berlin, Libr. Sin. 1238, Cohn 496, and from the *Imperial encyclopedia* (1726), Chen Menglei 17. 118, 8b. A trachea heart is also found in John of Arderne's *The art of medicine and surgery*, published after 1420, in the Royal library, Stockholm, Sudhoff 1915, 129, Pl. 4. The circulation man in the Pruefening five-picture series in figure 17 on page 28 is

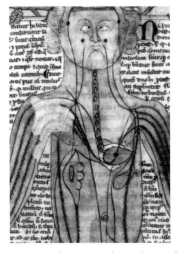 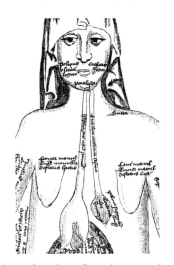

Fig.116. *Circulation man* from the Bodleian Ashmolean five-picture series, 1292, and Johannes de Ketham, *Pregnant woman*, 15th century.

without lungs too; the trachea leads directly to the base of the heart. Further examples of fourteenth-and fifteenth-century trachea hearts can be found in Ketham's *Fasciculus medicinae* Pl. 7, 8, 11, 12, see figure 116. The oesophagus leads to a configuration which is supposed to represent the stomach, but is, in fact, a copy of a hazelnut heart (see also figure 22 on page

32). For Ketham, see also note 65 and figure 113 on page 158. An idea of how little the illustrators (or the authors) understood of the texts to be illustrated can be gauged from the depiction of the trachea of the Bodleian-Ashmolean circulation man (manuscript 399), see figure 116). The rings of cartilage, which Galen (*On the usefulness of the parts of the body* 7.1.337) clearly described as semi-circular reinforcements of the tube, are represented in this drawing of the trachea not as running transversally, as in Donatello's trachea in figure 56 on page 68, but 'projected' as small rings on its outer wall.

74   For the Etruscan mirror, see Gladigow 352.

75   The three pairs are the two venae pulmonales dextrae, the two venae pulmonales sinistrae, and the arteriae pulmonales dextra and sinistra, Spalteholtz-Spanner 740. Dryander 39, Vesalius 64, 3-4, Eustachius 15. 4. For Casserio, see Singer 1957, fig.94. In dissecting a body, one can go a step further and leave the liver or the stomach attached, separated from the heart and lungs by the diaphragm, but attached to the heart by large blood vessels. 'Ligaments' probably refers to a part of the diaphragm, see figure 58 on page 70. For the autopsy report on Pope Alexander v, see Singer 1955, 94.

76   For the large, contemporary polyvisceral ex-votos in Bavaria and Tyrol, see Regnault 147. The depiction of Saint Ansanus in figure 60 on page 71 is in the Sant' Agnese basilica in Rome. Saint Ansanus is one of the early martyr saints. In 1910, Alice Kemp-Welch published a brief article devoted to him. In the beginning of the fourth century, he came to Siena, where he preached, baptized and wrought miracles. During the reign of the Emperor Diocletian, having been repeatedly tortured, he was boiled in oil and then beheaded round about 305. A chapel in Castel Vecchio was dedicated to him in 1107. He became the first patron saint of Siena. Towards the end of the middle ages, he disappeared into the background, partly because other patron saints of Siena had become more prominent, particularly Saint Bernardinus and Saint Catherine. Ansanus' depictions show him being boiled in oil (Kaftal 1952, fig.59) or being beheaded (*ibid.* fig.60). He is also

depicted with a variety of attributes, with a date palm (*ibid.* fig.56), as a baptizer with a pitcher (*ibid.* fig.57), and with a heart or with a trachea-lung-heart-liver specimen. It is conceivable that this attribute of Saint Ansanus refers to 'some legend of a horrible martyrdom, but none such appears to have been discovered' (Kemp-Welch 338). It is more plausible, however, to interpret his trachea-lung-heart-liver attribute as a sign of a miraculous curing of a heart ailment or some other internal complaint through his intervention. Similar specimens were still being encountered by Regnault in the 1920s as ex-votos in churches in Bavaria and the Tyrol region as thanks for the curing of internal disorders (see figure 59 on page 71). Ansanus is shown with an isolated heart in his hand in the San Bartolommeo a Quarata in Bagno a Ripoli (Kaftal 1952, 23e), on a panel by the Master of Signa (fifteenth century) in the Museo civico, Empoli, and possibly on a fresco by Francesco d'Antonio di Bartolommeo, about 1425, in the San Niccolo, Florence. For depictions of Saint Ansanus with a trachea-lung-heart-liver specimen see Kaftal 1986, 72, fig.68, Kaftal 1978, 50, fig.65, Marle 222, fig.137, Kemp-Welch figs a and c. The last-named considers this attribute to be a late echo of polyvisceral preparations used by the Etruscan haruspices (see also figures 9 on page 19 and 57 on page 69).

77 San Clemente, Rome, mosaic in the apse, near to the base of the cross. A red flame emerges from the mouth of the vase, Anthony Pl. 241, 228. A heart-icon shaped pitcher appears on a Coptic clavis from the third century, Forrer 1893, Pl. 8.6.

78 For the heart as the abode of a loved one in twelfth-century courtly poetry, see Ertzdorff *passim*. Hartmann von Aue (1321-1322): 'der sol si schuetten in ein vaz: / das ist ein herze ane haz'. Almost a century later, we find these lines in a poem by Walther von Grieven (384. 19-20): 'und tun die in ein reines vass / Ich meine in ein hertz on hass'. This was probably the source for the occurrence of this theme in later German literature.

79 The painted wooden sculpture of Saint Ansanus is by Francesco di Valdambrino, in the SS. Simone e Giuda, Lucca.

Bandinelli's *Venus* appeared in *The pray of Cupid and Apollo*, engraved by Antonio Salamanca, Rome 1545, Louvre, Paris. A pitcher heart like that of Saint Ansanus is also to be found in the hand of a late fifteenth-century Spanish wood-carving of Saint Catherine in the Santa Maria la Real, Medina del Campo, Bianchi 224. Although Saint Ansanus is depicted more frequently with a trachea-lung-heart specimen as an attribute, he was also occasionally shown, by Sodoma amongst others, as a baptizer carrying a pitcher, see *Bibliotheca sanctorum*, s.v. *Ansano di Siena* en Kaftal 1952, 23, fig.57. For Saint Ansanus, see also note 76. The conjunction of pitcher, heart and soul is clear, for example, in an engraving by Cornelis Galle (1576-1650), *Christ as the fisher of souls with the heart as the float* (see figure 117). The pitcher heart of Ansanus bears a strong

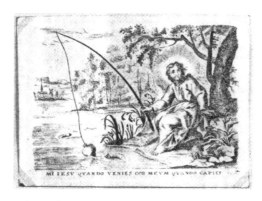

Fig.117. Cornelis Galle, *Christ*, with a pitcher heart symbolising the soul, 17th century.

resemblance to the pitcher heart of a seventeenth-century angel by Artus Quellin (school of), in the church of SS. Peter and Paul, Malines, which portrays the examination of conscience by probing the heart with a stick, Knipping 1. 141, see figure 118. We come across this metaphor in emblems of Georgette de Montenay (82), Roemer Visscher (3.45) and Julius Zincgref 87. In one of Montenay's emblems (15) the pot is compared to the heart: 'Comme les pots se sechent au soleil, aussi les coeurs des pervers s'endurcissent'. Aside from a (flaming) heart, Caritas also had a (flaming) pot as attribute. See notes 38 and 39. The Petrarchan heart appeared on the title page of the *Sonetti* published by Gabriel Giolito, Venice

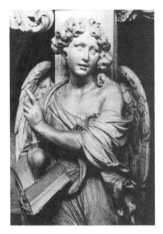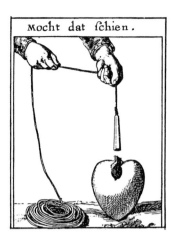

Mocht dat fchien.

Fig.118. Arthus Quellin's angel probing one's heart, about 1660, and one of Roemer Visscher's hearts, 1614.

1544, see Essling 1. 109. The heart-shaped vase is from *Il Petrarca*, published by Jean de Tournes, Lyons 1550. The concept that the poet's loved one dwells in his heart can already be found in twelfth-century courtly literature.

80 Hildegard of Bingen, a twelfth century abbess, already called the heart a little house in which the soul dwells, Bietenholz 19. On the same page: 'Another image portrays the heart as the chalice holding the sacred blood from the wound of christ's side. This chalice actually constitutes the core of one of the most important mythological tales of the early Middle Ages: Parsifal's quest for the Holy grail. Here we must remember that the association of the heart and the chalice came to Europe from Egypt, where the tradition of a very similar vessel in connection with the legend of Joseph of Arimathea, who supposedly brought the chalice of the Last Supper with him when he started his Gospel-spreading journeys to France and England in the first century.'

Large pitcher hearts also occur in, for example, an engraving by Hendrick Goltzius, *Christ as the example of virtuousness*, 1578, Sellink 1991-1992, fig.65 and on the title page of *Imagines et figurae bibliorum*, by Hendrik Barrefelt, published by Plantijn in 1584. For the popularity of heart symbolism in the seventeenth century, see also note 115. The illustrations in figure 63 are from Velde's *Openhertighe herten* (his first name is

166

unknown), Antoine Sucquet's *Den wegh des eewich levens* (516) and Etienne Luzuic's *Cor Deo devotum, passim.* Other illustrations of such large, 'habitable-hearts-with-chimneypiece' in Knipping 1. 136. Emblem books with heart symbolism are, for example, the compilations by Otto van Veen (1608 and 1615) and Van Haeften (1629). The largest pitcher hearts are to be found in the twenty copper plates of roughly A4 size by Martin Baes, from the school of Wierix, which appeared, for instance, in the various editions of Luzuic's *Le coeur devot* (1626). Latin translations appeared in 1627 and 1628. See also Knipping 1.3 and *passim.*

81   *Mortifiement*, see Lyna *passim.* The original is in the Staatliches Kupferstich Kabinett, Berlin, manuscript 566.

82   In Alciatus' emblem, we see a tree bearing indistinct fruit. The epigram reads: 'Fert folium linguae, fert poma simillima cordi', Henkel 236. Camerarius 1. 44. Also Junius 31.

83   Saint Augustine on an altar piece with the *Legend of Saint Ursula* by the Master of the Ursula legend from the 1480s in the Groeninge museum in Bruges and a panel by the Master of the Spes nostra, Rijksmuseum, Amsterdam. A similar peach-like heart in the hands of Saint Augustine appears on a panel of the Master of Alkmaar, illustration in *Middeleeuwse kunst der noordelijke Nederlanden*, catalogue of an exhibition in the Rijksmuseum, Amsterdam 1958, 90. Visscher, *Lootsmans water*, 3. 51. The spherical, peach-like hearts had already appeared a number of years earlier (1611) in Rollenhagen's emblems, 39, 43, 65, 79.

84   Galen, *On anatomical procedures* 7. 7. 605-607, Singer 1956, 180, Harris 269. Aristotle, *Parts of animals* 3. 4. 366, Peck 241: 'in man (the heart) inclines slightly to the left side' and *History of animals* 1. 17, Peck 65: 'its position is somewhat over towards the left, inclining slightly from the division of the breasts towards the left breast'. Rhazes was more explicit: 'The heart is placed in the middle of the thorax, but its tapered point inclines towards the left', Koning 63. For the Pruefening heart in figure 66, see figure 17 on page 28 and note 29. The second

heart is from the Caius circulation man, manuscript 190/223, Gonville and Caius college, Cambridge. For the Persian Mansur heart, see note 30. The post-mortem heart is from a late fourteenth-century manuscript of Guy de Chauliac, Bibliotheque de la faculte de medecine, 184, fol. 142r, Singer 1955 Pl. 29. The heart from Gregor Reisch's *Margarita philosophica* (Freiburg 1503) was published by Choulant 127. A unilateral indentation in the outline of the heart is also visible in the third heart in figure 22 on page 32. For Mondeville's text, Bos 90. 310: 'L'acuite de lui (c'est la pointe desous) se decline aucun poi vers la partie du pis senestre, si com dit le Philosophe ou .1. des hystoires des bestes, en la fin du .6. chapitre'.

85   Round about 1500, a *Madonna della misericordia* was carved in marble in the workshop of Gagini, holding such a one-sided concave heart in her hand, Bianchi 127. Saint Catharine is holding a comma heart (with the tip to the right) in a marble relief by the school of Gagini in the church of San Domenico

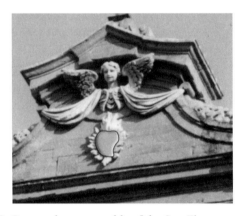

Fig.119. Comma heart on gable of the San Firenze monastery in Florence, 18th century.

in Taggia dating from circa 1500, Bianchi 127. The heart with a single concave side and a pronounced swing of the tip to the left was still being encountered in the eighteenth century, one example being Francesco del Rosso's decoration on the gable of the San Firenze monastery in Florence, see figure 119.

Occasionally the point of the heart is inclined towards the right; this is apparently due to a misunderstanding by the artist about the interpretation of left and right in a frontal rendering of the body: as seen from the spectator's viewpoint or from that of the figure represented. The present study follows the conventions of antomical works in using the terms 'right' and 'left' to indicate the direction as seen from the body in question.

86   The ivy leaf-shaped vertebrae and sacrum is from the fourteenth-century five-picture series in the *Codex Trivulziano* (Belloni figs 3 and 4). An ivy leaf-shaped urine bladder appears in a zodiac-man from *Margarita philosophica* (1503), Pl. 3v. A fifteenth-century Amor, with a waisted heart, is reproduced in Gombrich fig.151. Ivy-leaves are still common in water- and printers' marks, see Piccard *passim* and Davies *passim*.

87   The *Bundesgartenschau* was held in Gelsenkirchen, Germany from 19 April to 5 October 1997.

88   Mesue 1. 34, Pagel 1893, 33. Aristotle, *Parts of animals* 3, 4, 666b, Peck 1945, 239 and *History of animals* 1, 17, 496a, Peck 65. For Chauliac, see Wallner 1964, 112. Rufus of Ephesus, a predecessor of Galen from the first century, wrote that the heart is shaped like a pine-cone and terminates in a peak (Harris 264); elsewhere, he refers to it as a sharp point (Harris 265).

89   The old, pine-cone heart without a dip coexisted for a long time with the new, scalloped shape; relatively late examples can be found in the Persian five-picture series (see note 30), and on 'ancient' anatomical drawings from the fourteenth and fifteenth centuries, printed in Venice in 1491 (Ketham, see fig.116 on page 162 and notes 65 and 73). See also Schott Pl. 1, fig.2. The Peyligk heart in figure 49 was published in the 1499 edition of the *Compendium*, that in figure 50 on page 60 in the 1516 edition, Herrlinger 66.

90   For Fra Angelico's *Caterina da Siena ed altri Beati Domenicani*, National gallery, London, Bianchi 183, Pl. 15. See also Fra Angelico's painting dating from circa 1430, mentioned in note

42. In a later work by the Dutch painter Joost van Cleve, another Dominican (probably Hendrik Suso) offers his (scalloped) heart to the Virgin. The same scene can be found in a painting by an unknown master from the Southern Netherlands, dating from the first half of the sixteenth century, in the Louvre, Paris, Knipping 1. 133, fig.88. Fiorenzo di Lorenzo's Antony is in the Pinacoteca of Perugia, Kleinschmidt 98, fig.56. For the sculpture of Saint Catherine, see Bianchi 225. The pine-cone-shaped heart can be found in watermarks up to the beginning of the sixteenth century, Briquet 3. 4240, 4241, 4246 etc. For the Tibetan temple decorations, see Eschmann figs 13, 37. See also note 35.

91   For the illustrations in figure 74 see Clark 19073v, Saunders Pl. 64.1, and *Gray's anatomy*, fig.10.28 and 1475. Also: Schott *passim*, and Harris 85. In his *Fabrica* (1543, 6. 8), Vesalius still calls the heart pine-cone-shaped and its base round. The contour of the base of an excised heart is sometimes frayed as, for example, in the heart in the centre figure of the Benetton hearts in figure 73 on page 83, the Mesoamerican hearts in figure 6 on page 11, the Etruscan hearts in figure 11 on page 22. This results from the sloppy way in which the hearts were removed from the chest cavity. In these cases, one or more pieces of the large blood vessels still adhere to the heart base.One gets a very good idea of this by looking at figure 45 on page 52. An example of such a frayed heart base as a saintly attribute can be seen in the hand of Sodoma's Saint Antony in Siena, Kleinschmidt fig.84. See also notes 20, 27, 30, 32 and 36.

92   Nahum Zenil, *Ex-voto. Self portrait with the Virgin of Guadelupe* appeared on the cover of *Art journal* 57. 1, Spring 1998. It features a picture of the heart, obviously derived from an anatomy book, into which a knife has been plunged. The composition conjures up associations with the pierced heart of Saint Augustine. Alain Miller's painting is in the Saatchi collection, London, illustrated in *Sensation* 125. The first picture of figure 73 appeared in the major Dutch newspapers on 19 September 1995, the second on the cover of the *New scientist* on 8 June 1996, the third in the *Spectator* on 19 July 1997, 22 and the fourth in the Dutch morning paper *Algemeen dagblad* on 9

September 1997. The Benetton advertisement appeared on European billboards and in newspapers in the first half of 1996.

94 A first version of this study on Spiegel's *Antrum Platonicum* was published in *Oud Holland* in 1960. In the present, considerably extended version, I have taken into account the subsequent reactions, notably the article by Thiel. For Spiegel, see Buisman *passim*, Israel 567-568 and McGee 127-129, 239-252. For the dating of Spiegel's text see Zijderveld and Thiel. Spiegel (or: Spieghel) advocated his linguistic principles in his *Twe-spraack van de Nederduitse letterkunst* ('Dialogue on Dutch literature', 1584). There was regular contact between scholars and artists in Haarlem and those in Leyden (18 miles) and Amsterdam (16 miles). In neoplatonic ethics, self-knowledge and its symbol, the looking-glass, plays an important role, for example, in Plato's *Alcibiades* 1, 133c.

95 The quotations are from Verwey 160 and Knuvelder 390.

96 The allegory of the cave is described in Plato's *Republic*, Book 7. Hirschmann 82. The print is signed: *C.C. Harlemensis Inv. J. Sanredam sculpsit, Henr. Hondius excudit 1604*.

97 Mander, *Grondt* 7. 45-46 fol. 32v. 33r, Miedema 197-198, 527. See Appendix 1.

98 Veenstra's edition of *Hertspiegel* 3, 63-89. For the Dutch text, see Appendix 2.

99 Mander, *Schilder-boeck* fol. 293r. 11-13: 'een eerste Weerelt oft gulde Eeuwe / welck stuck noch is t'Amsterdam by den Const-verstandighen Heer Hendrick Louwersz. Spieghel' and fol. 288v. 32-33: 'den Const-lievenden Heer Hendrick Louwersz. Spieghel t' Amsterdam', Miedema 1994, 3-7. Mander mentions four paintings which were in Spiegel's collection, Greve 294.

100 Thiel 316.

101 Thiel (314) situated Ruyschestein along the river Amstel, past

the present-day Kalfjeslaan. 'Daar hielt Apollo feest; Euterpes Orgel schoon / stont an de ooster-muijr; daar vooren in den thoon / Arion op den Dolphijn vroolijk zatt en speelde' [There held Apollo revels; Euterpe's organ stood elegantly against the east wall; displayed in front of it Arion on the dolphin cheerfully sat and played.] *Hertspiegel* 7. 75-77, Veenstra 178, Thiel 314, 316, 317, fig.2, note 25. The *Arion* print was discussed by Thiel, who dated it between 1589 and 1591. It has emblematic characteristics similar to the *Antrum* print. He assumed that the Arion print was probably copied from a painting by Cornelisz, also conceived by Spiegel. Spiegel's town house, which was built about 1600 on the Singel 140-142 in Amsterdam, is still called 'The dolphin'.

102 The sources of Spiegel's story of Arion are described by Veenman. Spiegel was not the first person to use Arion astride the dolphin as a personal device. Prior to him, in the 1540s, Johann Oporinus, printer of Vesalius' *Fabrica*, had chosen the theme for his printer's mark. And in 1533, two years after the appearance of Alciatus' *Emblemata*, the German printer, Georg Rhau, also used Arion on the dolphin as his mark, Grimm 219.

103 The passage is from *Hertspiegel* 7. 89-99, Veenstra 178-179. See Appendix 3.

104 'Zoet ende zacht moetse [de dueghd] zijn isse natuurlijk: maar Platoos / spelonk, verkeerd verstand ende wennis is alleen in de weegh'. The letter was incorporated for the first time in the *Hertspiegel* edition of 1694, 121-130. Intellectuals of the time must have been familiar with the 'symbolic values of the cave, derived from a tradition that originates in Homer's epic *Odyssey* and that is given its most striking expression in Plato's myth of the cave, where slaves, chained at the bottom of a pit, take shadows on the wall for reality. For Plato, as for Homer, the cave represents illusion, ignorance, possession by the passions, primitivism, simplicity, life at an animal level, privation, austerity, darkness of the soul. A number of these connotations are sometimes given a positive significance, whenever primitivism and simplicity are considered virtues.

(...) The prisoner's progress up from the earthly womb parallels the basic Greek (and Judaic) idea of man's origins, struggling up from autochthonous beginnings (...) into the free air. From darkness, he rises into light, moving from low to high', Weinberg 223.

105 The difference between Spiegel's *Antrum* and Plato's account can in part be explained by the influence of a similar theme from Aristotle which appeared in his lost dialogue *De philosophia*, but which is known to us by a quotation in Cicero's *De natura deorum* (2.95): 'If there were beings who had always lived beneath the earth, in comfortable, well-lit dwellings, decorated with statues and pictures and furnished with all the luxuries enjoyed by persons thought to be supremely happy, and who thought they had never come forth above the ground had learnt by report and by hearsay of the existence of certain deities or divine powers; and then if at some time the jaws of the earth were opened and they were able to escape from their hidden abode and to come forth into the regions which we inhabit; when they suddenly had sight of the earth and the seas and the sky, and came to know of the vast clouds and mighty winds, and beheld the sun (...) surely they would think that the

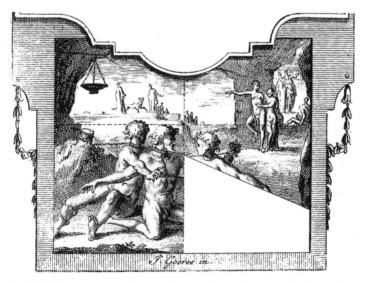

Fig.120. Plato's cave, an illustration in Hendrik Spiegel's *Hieroglifica* which appeared in the 18th-century *Hertspiegel* editions.

gods exist and that these mighty marvels are their handiwork'. The inhabitants of Aristotle's cave are more comfortably situated than the prisoners in Plato's cave. Vlaming, the editor of the eighteenth-century editions of the *Hertspiegel*, added a few emblems engraved by Goeree. One of these is a more accurate representation of Plato's text (174), see figure 120.

It is an open question whether these *Hieroglifica*, which have appeared in all *Hertspiegel* editions since Wetstein's, can actually be attributed to Spiegel. In the Rijksmuseum print collection, there is a large, unsigned wood-cut from which the *Hieroglifica* in the 1694 edition are copied. The woodcuts are accompanied by the same verses found in the *Hieroglifica*. The *Andere hieroglifica*, which first appeared in the Vlaming editions, were probably not the work of Spiegel.

Spiegel's print shows a greater similarity to Aristotle's description than to Plato's. Also, the figures standing on the wall bear more resemblance to the statues decorating the dwellings of Aristotle than to Plato's low puppet-show stage. The splitting of the earth in Spiegel's text recalls the opening of the 'jaws of the earth' in Cicero. The contents of Cicero's book were generally known to intellectual circles in Spiegel's time. Pease lists more than 70 editions before 1600. There was also a French translation (Paris 1581).

Obviously not aware of the original engraving of the *Antrum* by Saenredam, Jong illustrated his 1930 edition of the first three books of the *Hertspiegel* with a smaller copy after the original engraving. This copy appeared for the first time in the 1694 edition of the *Hertspiegel*, where it was inserted as an illustration in Book 3, between pages 32 and 33. Wetstein, editor of the 1694 edition, states in his preface that he added the print of Plato's cave as an illustration to the text. It was engraved by Jos Mulder after the original by Jan Saenredam. Wetstein apparently knew that the original print was published by Spiegel: 'Verder om de Hertspiegel te verlichten, hebben wij hier ingevoegt een print van het hol van Plato, van Spiegel zelf voor henen uit gegeven'. – (To throw further light on the Hertspiegel, we have here inserted a print of Plato's cave, previously published by Spiegel himself). The verse accompanying the print has also been cited from the 1694 edition by Jong in 1930. Knipping (1. 62) illustrated his book with the eighteenth-century copy of the *Antrum Platonicum* from the Vlaming edition of 1723 and wrongly attributed this to Saenredam. Buisman (22, note 2) also refered to the illustration of Plato's cavern in *Hertspiegel*; he dated it (incorrectly) 1605.

106 Bartsch (39) refered to the print as a 'piece emblematique'.

107 Jong 135.73: 'It cannot be seen on the plate that the cave has the shape of a human heart'. Knipping 1. 131: ' Spiegel would, for example, have liked to have seen that Plato's cave assume the shape of a human heart, because it had such a striking likeness to it, but neither his plate cutter or drawer thought that this would be possible, or because he set himself against such a literary prank, the print, which had to illustrate the Hertspiegel, fulfils in no way the poet's wish'. ('Spiegel zou bijvoorbeeld gaarne gezien hebben, dat de grot van Platoon de vorm van een mensenhart zou aannemen, omdat ze daarvan zo'n treffend beeld geleek, doch of zijn plaatsnijder of tekenaar er geen kans toe zag, of dat hij zich verzette tegen zo'n literaire stoutigheid, de prent, die de Hertspiegel illustreren moet, vervult de dichterswens in geen geval').

108 For Paaw as an anatomist, see Heckscher s.v. *Paauw* and fig.2, Plates 3.3 and 33-40. Also Prinsen and Lunsingh Scheurleer *passim*.

109 Paaw note 8 and note 43: Cor innata cupiditate aerem expetit, ut ejus ope fervidum suum innatum temperet calorem, trahit autem eum non per septem ventriculis interjectum, verum mediante arteria venosa e pulmone. Authoris [i.e. *Vesalius*] verba videntur hac in parte dubia paululum quum dicant: *Et in sinistrum ipsius ventriculum magnam sanguinis copiam a dextro alliciens.* non enim trahit sanguinem e dextro ventriculo immediate, sed prius pulmoni infusum.

110 *Hippocratic writings* 12. See also note 7. This paragraph and figure 81 are derived from Lind's facsimile edition of Vesalius' *Epitome*, Hofmann *passim*. For Leonardo's sketch, see Clark 3. 19112r.

111   Galen, *On anatomical procedures* 7. 11. 623, Singer 1956, 188. Galen also disputes with Aristotle on this point and writes that the chambers 'do not differ according to size', *On anatomical procedures* 7.10.618, Singer 1956, 186. For Avicenna's quotation, see Koning 688.

112   Vesalius' *Fabrica* 6, fig.3, Saunders 180, Pl. 64.1, Paaw 4.8 and 4.9. One is bound to conclude from the addition of the vertical apex line in the second state of the print that it was also absent from Cornelisz' painted original.

113   Quoted from Siegel (37, 40, 161), who also cites Hippocrates: '... respiration (*rhipizesthai*, literally, fanning the fire) serves the principle of indwelling heat [in the left ventricle] ...' *Hippocratic writings* 347-351, Deichgraeber 9, Plato's *Timaeus* 62a, also Leboucq 28, Singer 1956, 251, note 152, Eijk 11, 18. Hippocrates: 'the heart, being the hottest part in a person, holds the breath (...) if you light a fire inside a room when no wind is blowing in, the flame moves, sometimes more, sometimes less. Also a lighted lamp moves in the same way', *Fleshes*, 4, Potter 142-143. Aristotle, *Parts of animals, passim*, also Harris 125, 170, 171. In contrast to the Hippocratic tradition and to Galenic theory, Aristotle considered the blood in the right chamber the hottest. See also note 27. For Aristotle, see Harris 125, 135, for Galen, see Harris 304, 305, 340. See also note 132.

114   The flame flaring towards the tunnel's exit recalls to mind the qoutation from Hippocrates' *Fleshes* in note 113. Galen, *On the doctrines of Hippocrates and Plato* 3. 1. 28ff, Harris 304, 305, 273, 275, Singer 1956, 184, 251, Siegel 161 and May 292, Flint 18. Hieronymo Manfredi's *Anathomia*: '(the heart) is pyramidal, that is in the form of a flame', Singer 1955, 122, 126. In his *Grande chirurgie*, Guy de Chauliac compares the heart with the hearth of the body ('c'est comme un four de feu a tout le corps', Nicaise 33). Paaw note 8: 'Sunt hi velut thalami vitae humanae, horum qui dexter capacior multo sinistroque in quo praeparatio, uti sinistro perfectio fit vitalis sanguinis'. In accordance with the 'physiological' symbolism, in Book 4 of *Hertspiegel*, Spiegel describes the left chamber of the heart as the location of the

higher, critical and directing functions (Apollo and Clio), dividing the inhabitants of our inner life into masters and servants (244-250). Flint 28, Vesalius' *Fabrica*, Praefatio.

115 For the two kinds of love, see *Hertspiegel* 7. 414-450, Veenstra 194-196. *Das Buch Extasis* was published in Cologne between 1573 and 1576, foreword *Apodixe* 273. In an emblem by Georgette de Montenay (1571), *Amor divinus* holds the globe: without love the world collapses, see figure 121. For the

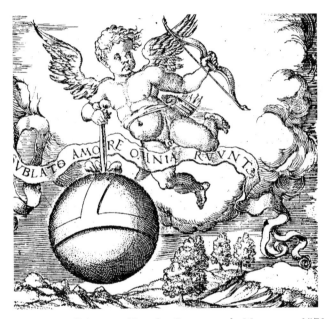

Fig.121. *Amor divinus*, emblem by Georgette de Montenay, 1571.

complexity of the Caritas concept in the late middle ages, see Freyhan *passim*, specifically 68, 69, 73-77, 85 and notes 3 and 4. Saint Augustine: Caritas est nexus quo homines invicem sibi et Deo connectantur (...) Caritas est virtus quae, cum nostra affectio est rectissima, conjugit nos Deo, qua eum diligimus (...) Caritas dicitur amor Dei et proximi. (...) Caritas, *amor proximi*, is valuable only for God's sake (...) is valueless, even reprehensible, without the major quality, *amor Dei*, (...) the two forms of Caritas were really inseparable. A scene typifying *amor proximi* would therefore imply the presence of the other side of virtue, *amor*

Dei (...). For the quotes from Augustine, see Burnaby 116, also 117, 129, 149, 150 and for similar passages from Saint Thomas Aquinas 268 ff. In the encyclopaedic *Breviari d'amor* (end of the thirteenth century), the distinction between the two types of love is expressed as follows: 'La sobirana taula premieira es d'amor de Dieu, l'autra d'amor de prueime', Laske-Fix 52. Francesco Barberino in his *Documenti d'amore* permits Amor to preside over a group of twelve virtues. For Barberino, see page 44 and note 46. For the split between sacred and profane love in the sixteenth century, see Yates *passim*. Coornhert 1586, 7. 7. Corrozet 180, Henkel 1765. The motto is *Amour accompaignee de vertu* and the epigram runs: 'Quand ces deux se treuuent ensemble Par effect, et non en paincture, Tout s'en porte mieulx, ce me semble, Selon la reigle de droicture'. Such an Amor, as a heathen deity, standing on a column had appeared earlier on Jacopo Pontormo's *Joseph with Jacob in Egypt* (1518?), National gallery, London. Also in an emblem in Alciati's Paris 1542 edition of *Emblematum libellus*, Amor is standing on a (lower) pillar. In the middle ages, deities or heathen idols were often represented on columns, see, e.g. Laborde Pl. 9, 11, 18, 19, 22, 38, 39, 80, 81, 87. Montenay 45, Henkel 1764: 'Par vray amour tout l'Vniuers est faict, Et par luy seul tout est entretenu: Par luy aussi tout conduict et parfaict, Et de luy seul aussi tout sustenu. Qui a ceci cognoistre est paruenu, En admirant ceste bonte divine, Reiettera ce fol qu'on bande nu, Cause de mal, et toute ruine'. Divine love, represented by a halo-ed Amor, occurs repeatedly in the *emblemata amatoria* from the early seventeenth century, for example in those of Otto van Veen (*Amoris divini emblemata*, 1615), of Etienne Luzuic (*Le coeur devot*, 1626) and of Benedictus van Haeften (*Schola cordis*, 1629), all entirely based on conceits of the heart. In Otto van Veen's book there is an emblem (61) with the title *Uyt liefde komen alle deugden* (all virtues stem from love), and according to emblem 89, Love stands above the Virtues:

> Amour des vertus la plus grande
> Teint entre elles le lieu premier
> Et seul dessus toute la bande.

Amor as Divine love also plays a leading role in the most popular of the Jesuit emblem books, Herman Hugo's *Pia*

Desideria, Antwerp 1624.

116   For *Diffidentia Dei* see Philip Galle 38. As a young man, Goltzius worked for Galle in Antwerp prior to setting up his own atelier in Haarlem. Similar money-pouches can be seen in *The misuse of prosperity* (as Riches), a series of woodcuts by Cornelis Antonisz., dated 1546 (Armstrong fig.25c), in Hendrik Pot's *The miser* in the Reinisches Landesmuseum, Bonn, in engravings by Dirck Coornhert, Veltman fig.10, 17, 21, in Pieter Bruegel's drawings *Avaritia* (1556), *Elck* (1558), in his engraving *Battle between piggy banks and strong boxes* (1570s), and in Hendrick Goltzius' *Danae* (1603) in a putto's hand. Sluijter fig.279. Speaking about this painting, Karel van Mander calls it a 'stick purse', *Schilderboeck* 286r. Such a purse contains a number of separate compartments for the various denominations of coins and was held by a short stick. The money-purse as attribute of Avaritia already appears in the middle ages, Liebeschuetz 53.238. For avaritia forming 'the ideal counterpart to the misericordia side of Caritas', see Freyhan 81. Also *Blockbuecher* 43a, fig.4.34.

117   The Fool in figure 90 is from Cats 24. The fool, together with his sausage-like bauble, is regularly found in Cats' emblems. For *Hans Worst*, see *Woordenboek der Nederlandsche taal*, 1900, 5, 2117-2118. Martin Luther used the word in a pamphlet (1541) against Duke Heinrich von Braunschweig-Wolfenbuettel, Hohenemser note 12.2. The Fool on the *Antrum* wall has the sausage hanging on his stick as if it were a fishing rod. The fool in a painting by Adriaen Rombouts, *Fool of a Brussels chamber of rhetoric* (1657) is holding just such a stick with a sausage-like appendage, see Vandenbroeck fig.62. Somewhat earlier (1561), Philip Galle in Haarlem had engraved a *Tabula Cebetis* after a design by Frans Floris. His *Prosopographia* dates from about 1590. It is a small iconological thesaurus of unusual and sophisticated personifications, and was used internationally by artisans and poets (Sellink 1997, 132, also 94ff). In his Foreword, Galle wrote that, 'at present (...) Christian inventions are more in vogue and held in higher esteem'.

118   For *Maiestas,* see Galle 23.

119 For *Sanitas*, see Galle 10. *Hertspiegel* 6. 530, Veenstra 170. See also note 127. In *Wellevenskunst*, a hierarchical outline of his ethics, which was first published in the 1694 edition of Hertspiegel, Spiegel drew a distinction between body and soul in dealing with emotions, virtues, and vices, adding that the pleasures of the flesh are natural and healthy, as long as they lead only to simple release of the need for sustenance and therefore they comply with reason. But if one feels Lust, then it brings on bodily ruination, is unnatural, and makes man a slave to lechery. ('Natuurlijk ende heilzaam is ende blijft de lijf-lust, zo langh die alleenlik strekt tot simpele boeting van noodruft tot ons onderhout ende alzo ghehoorzaamt zij de reden. Maar voltmen de *Lust*, zo ghedijt zy tot lijfs-onheil, wert onnatuurlijk, ende maakt den mensch een slaaf van de wel-lust'). For the well-being of the body, see *Hertspiegel* 6. 499-515, Veenstra 169-170.

120 A number of copies have been made of the Niklaus Deutsch mural, but only those dating from the eighteenth century have survived (Vignau fig.72). A large etching by Maarten van Heemskerck, *The dangers of human ambition* (1549) also makes one think about Spiegel's cave. It shows a variety of figures walking along a narrow footplank, situated high above the spectators, and connecting two walls. One or two of them fall of it down to the ground below, Veldman 1977, 53 and note 109. Van Heemskerck was perhaps inspired by a woodcut included in the French translation (Paris 1546) of Francesco Colonna's *Hypnerotomachia Poliphili*, which was first published in Venice in 1499. In the latter, some of the figures are falling off a footplank-style bridge between two sections of a cave, Colonna 237. (There are no human figures in the illustration of the original Italian edition.)

121 For the original Latin epigram, see Appendix 4; it was translated by Harm-Jan van Dam.

122 Thiel (315) identified the bent figure as Christ. A clue in this direction can also be found in the text of *Hertspiegel* (7. 304, Veenstra 189): 'door s'Heijllands hulp ontwijflijk hij geraakt tott tem-lusts zoete zeegh (...) te gaan den effen weegh'.

123   Limbo forms the first circle of hell and its inhabitants include the virtuous pagans, poets, philosophers and heroes of classical antiquity (Hall 100). Christ descended into hell during the period from his death to the resurrection (for biblical and other sources, see Kirschbaum 2, 322 and Male 224-226). We find this 'bending over attitude' of Christ in limbo in numerous post-medieval depictions, for example, in the basilica of the Holy martyrs in Cimitile, eighth century, in the Codex Helmstedtensis in Wolfenbuettel (1195), on a mural by Pietro Lorenzetti in the lower church of San Francesco in Assisi (1325-1330), in the bronze relief by Donatello on the pulpit in the S. Lorenzo in Florence (1460), in Dürer's woodcuts of the Passion (1510), and in his engraving of Christ's *Descent into hell* (1512), in Lucas van Leyden's engraving *Christ in limbo* (1521), in Antoni Wierix' engraving *Christ in limbo*, Wierix fig.17 and on the Bordelsholm altar by Brueggeman in Schleswig (1521). Schiller figs 102, 103, 104, 108, 110, 131, 139, 141, 146, 152, 156, 165, 166, 169. An example that may also have contributed to this image of Christ is the pit in Hans Holbein's woodcut *Christ as the light of the world* (about 1522), in which Plato, Aristotle and other pagan philosophers walk away from the light of the flaming lamp to which Christ draws attention, to fall into the abyss, Baetschmann fig.158.

124   *Hertspiegel* 6. 45, Veenstra 147. Spiegel's translation (*Cebetis des thebaenschen philosoophs tafereel*) and its synopsis (*Kebes tafereels kort begrip*) appeared for the first time in the *Hertspiegel* edition of 1615.

125   Matham's large print consists of three engravings, each measuring 66.5 x 41.7 cm. Thus, the complete depiction of this *Tabula* measures 66.5 x 125.1 cm., much larger than the *Antrum* print, which measures 14.8 x 25.2 cm. There is a much smaller copy of the Matham print, engraved by N.I. Visscher in 1640, and a later one with the same format engraved by Justus Danckerts. See Holstein under Matham 253.
Thiel (317) pointed out that the *Arion* print, with the *Antrum* and *Tabula* scenes, may have suggested the idea of a triptych to Spiegel. It is, however, no easy task to image a triptych in which the front of the two doors form a square (Arion) when

they are closed, while when they are opened the inside would present two oblong representations. But, of course, the choice of the poet's themes need not have been disturbed by such a mundane consideration.

126   *Hertspiegel* 6. 42-45: 'Het huijs vol schilderij, al beelt-schrift, sin-rijk, tuchtich; / Des voorzaals noorder want was heel, en al bemaalt / met Kebes tafereel, daar op zij ditt verhaalt'.
Spiegel is reminded by the muse Erato that he had commenced learning Greek thirteen years earlier. See Appendix 6. If we follow Zijderveld in assuming that this part of the book was written about 1600, Spiegel must have begun his study of Greek about 1587. The Goltzius print dates from 1592. The three engravings corresponding to the representations on these panels were created independently of the text, the *Arion* and *Tabula* prints, even before the corresponding passages in the *Hertspiegel* had been written. The *Antrum* print was created afterwards, but the original painting by Cornelisz was in Spiegel's possession. Schleier's book contains numerous illustrations of *Tabula* representations from the sixteenth and seventeenth centuries. Long before Spiegel, Erasmus described imaginary paintings in *Convivium religiosum* (1522). The latter, in his turn, in describing such paintings, had been inspired by Philostratos' *Imagines* (about AD 300), Schlueter *passim*. The oldest French translation of the *Tabula Cebetis* dates from 1529, the English from 1530 and the German, by Hans Sachs, from 1531. Warners *passim*, Fitzgerald *passim*.

127   *Hertspiegel* 6. 47ff. and Book 7 *passim*. See also note 119. Aside from Sanitas, other symbolical figures on the wall are derived from those out of the first ring of Tabula representations. So, the female figure with the same money-pouches appears as Fortuna in an early painting (1573) of the *Tabula* by an anonymous Northern Netherlandish master, in the Rijksmuseum, Amsterdam (81a, 3243) and in Goltzius' *Tabula* (see figure 93). In both paintings, we find a Bacchus figure and the symbols of Majesty.

128   *Hertspiegel* 6. 492-497, Veenstra 168-169, see Appendix 5.

129   For a summary of the ten types of people in the second ring of *Kebes tafereel*, see Spiegel's *Tabula Cebetis* in the 1615 *Hertspiegel* edition. A similar summary is included in *Hertspiegel* (6. 499-502), but it is arranged differently and is less complete than that appearing in *Kebes tafereel*: 'rich in medicine, in law, in knowledge of languages, mathematics, in schoolwise debate, in rhyming, in declamation, in rhetoric seems goodly'. A few lines further (6. 504), he summarizes these practitioners of science and art as university baccalaureates in the 'art', i.e. the liberal arts. *Hertspiegel* 6. 289-291, Veenstra 168. This citation is followed by the text contained in Appendix 5. Veenstra (64) incorrectly took the circular edge of the hat of the man standing near the entrance to the tunnel for a nimbus, and, accordingly, but incorrectly, took him to represent Jesus Christ.

130   The figure Fucata eruditio was also a model for Spiegel's False knowledge (False learning, False education) which stands on the wall of the *Antrum*, also with an open book. It is reminiscent of the Sibyl in Vergil's underworld. The undergound cave, extreme right in Goltzius' *Tabula Cebetis* (figure 93 on page 113), is apparently derived from the limbo caves, examples being those of Lucas van Leyden or of Albrecht Dürer, see note 123.

131   Other portraits of Spiegel at the age of 30, bearing a strong likeness, were published in the *Hertspiegel* editions of 1614 and

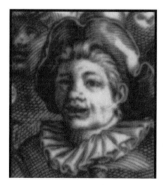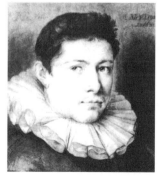

Fig.122. Portraits of Jacob Matham by Hendrick Goltzius, in the *Tabula*, and on a drawing, both from 1592.

1615. There is also a portrait of Spiegel amongst the *Archers of the Handboogdoelen* in Dirck Barendsz' portrait (1585) of the Amsterdam historical museum, Veenstra CXVII. Goltzius had pictured his pupil, Matham in his *Tabula,* see figure 122, Widerkehr 226. In the seventeenth century, it was not unusual for painters to include their own images in group portraits. It is not too far-fetched to suggest that Spiegel would have allowed himself to be depicted, also in a less flattering situation, in a scene of his own composition. Rembrandt portrayed himself as a sinner in the *Raising of the Cross* (circa 1633), and Jan Steen included himself in his paintings with great regularity (Jongh 43), also in less favourable poses.

132   Hippocrates: 'Man's intelligence, the principle which rules over the rest of the soul, is situated in the left chamber', Lloyd 351. The heart as the seat of mental and emotional activities is an opinion mainly attributable to the Aristotelian school, to Plato and others. Instead, Galen considered the heart only as seat of the *energeiai physicai* which principally concern the production of heat in the body, Siegel 143. Also Galen, *On the doctrines of Hippocrates and Plato* 3. 1. 32ff. See also note 113.
In a painting of the *Tabula Cebetis* from 1573 (see note 127), a tunnel also runs from the second ring to the top of the mountain.

133   These pendants are in the State museum, Cassel (*Tabula* GK 1176, *Underworld* GK 1177), Schleier figs. 45 and 46.
Nevertheless, there are perhaps reminiscences of the *Aeneid*. In Book 6, Aeneas descends into the Lower world. Spiegel describes the *Tabula* in Book 6 of the *Hertspiegel*. Aeneas was guided through the Lower world by the Cumaean Sibyl; in Spiegel's *Antrum,* the learned are addressed by a Sibyl-like woman. For the connections between the *Tabula Cebetis* and the Lower world of Vergil, see Schleier 120, note 306. There is also another Dutch painting depicting the *Tabula Cebetis* which Spiegel could have seen, see note 127.
The engraving by Goltzius (figure 93 on page 113) has many similarities with the two panels referred to in the text, both that in Cassel and in Amsterdam, although they too relate back to older examples (Boas 15). Another example was perhaps the

large engraving, composed of two sections, by Philip Galle after Frans Floris and dating from 1561, Velde P.134, fig.287. A later painting, dated 1624, by Joris van Schooten, in the Lakenhal museum in Leyden, could have been inspired by Galle's or Goltzius' engraving. Perhaps it was the unusual size of Goltzius' *Tabula Cebetis* engraving that provided Spiegel with the idea to decorate the entire north wall of the vestibule in his dream house (*Hertspiegel* 6. 42-44) with a mural devoted to this composition.

The concentric path of virtue to the top of the mountain in many *Tabula Cebetis* representations can be recognized in Dante's *Mountain of purgatory*, with paradise on top, impressively represented in Domenico di Michelino's fresco (1465) in Florence cathedral, see figure 123. Artists may have seen it and

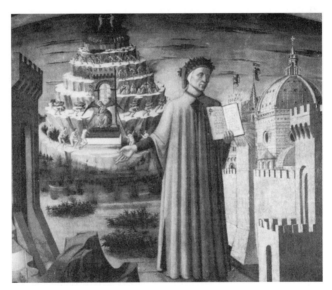

Fig.123. Domenico di Michelino, fresco, 1465, Florence cathedral.

it may have influenced their *Tabula* versions. (The *Tabula* text was, of course, unknown in Dante's time.) – At the rhetoricians festival held in Ghent from 12-23 June 1539, the Wynoxberghe company of actors presented a play in which the situation of one of the symbolical personages (who had the significant name of Frustrated heart) is compared with the occupant of the world's cave ('s waerelds speloncken'), Dis 330. 91.

134 Veenstra (70, i) doubted whether the hunchback was intended to represent Aesop, and decided that is was 'probably Socrates'. He did not advance any arguments for reaching this conclusion. Rightly or wrongly, programmatically or not (out of revenge for his difficult questions about demonstrating that the superior one did not reside per se in a beautiful body), Socrates was described, even in antiquity, as an ugly, untidy man with a big bald head, bulbous eyes, thick lips and a large fat belly, and he was compared to Silenus or to a satyr (Zanker 34, 36 and 348 note 54, and *passim*).

135 For Hendrik Niclaes and the *House of love* (Huis der liefde), see Fontaine Verwey *passim*. It considers the impact the House of love had in the Netherlands, Germany and England. For the (English) *Family of love*, see Ebel, Hitchcock and Moss. An illustration of a scalloped heart was frequently used at the end of the books by Hendrick Niclaes, Moss 38. For Plantin's (and Abraham Ortelius') membership, see Sabbe 75.

136 The representations and the text about the cordiform maps are derived from Kish. Fine's map was published under the title *Recens et integra orbis descriptio,* Honter's map *Orbis universalis descriptio* was published in his *Cosmographiae rudimentis*, Basle 1561.

137 Coornhert's *Hert-spiegel* was published in Amsterdam in 1632. This book, like Spiegel's *Hertspiegel* (and, for that matter, Niklaes' *Spegel*), can be regarded as late examples of a long series of medieval ethical tracts with the word *speculum* in the title, a large number of which appeared in the late fourteenth century and during the fifteenth century. There was even a *Spieghel dines herten* ('Mirror of your heart') written by an anonymous fifteenth-century author. This too contained virtuous instruction; man needs an internal mirror in order to know himself and one in which God can be reflected. Man has need of many virtues and must avoid many vices, so as to be able to find the right path to God. Thereby, the heart of man can serve as a house in which Jesus Christ dwells, Bange

passim. In an engraving by Goltzius, *Allegory of the necessity of prudence*, 1578, mankind is typified as a man looking at himself in a mirror, alive to the importance of self-knowledge. With the assistance of 'sensible judgement', he can receive divine grace and can be judged good enough to be received in heaven, Sellink 1991-1992, 152.

138 This is the last sentence of the relevant passage from *Hertspiegel*, see Appendix 2.

139 This sentence is the last of the passage from Mander, quoted on page 89. Spiegel's *Antrum*, which is also a symbol of the soul, heralds a fashion in heart symbolism which was to become extremely popular among Jesuit and Benedictine writers towards the middle of the seventeenth century, and which was closely associated with the convention of Amor and Anima. See also notes 80 and 115.

REFERENCES

Adelphus, Johannes, *Mondini de omnibus corporis interioribus membris anathomia*, Strasbourg 1513.

Albertus Magnus, *De animalibus*. Published by Hermann Stadler, Muenster 1916. (Beitraege zur Geschichte der Philosophie des Mittelalters 15).

Alcalde del Rio, H., Henri Breuil, Lorenzo Sierra, *Les cavernes de la region Cantabrique (Espagne)*, Monaco 1911. (Peintures et gravures murales des cavernes paleolithiques 3).

Alfredus Anglicus, see Baeumker.

Anjou, Rene of, see Lyna, see also Trenkler.

Anthony, E.W., *A history of mosaics*, New York 1968, reprint of the 1935 edition.

Aristotle, *The complete works*. The revised Oxford translation. Edited by Jonathan Barnes, 2 vols, Princeton, 1984, *On sleep*, 1.

Aristotle, *History of animals*. With an English translation by A.L. Peck. 3 vols, London 1965. (The Loeb classical library 437-439).

Aristotle, *De partibus animalium and De generatione animalium*. Translated with notes by D.M. Balme, Oxford 1972. (Clarendon Aristotle series).

Aristotle, *Parts of animals*. With an English translation by A.L. Peck, London 1937. (The Loeb classical library 323).

Aristotle, *Parva naturalia*. With a French translation and introduction by J. Tricot, Paris 1951.

Aristotle, *Vier Buecher ueber die Theile der Thiere*. Greek and German text with notes by A. Frantzius, Leipzig 1853.

Armstrong, C.M., *The moralizing prints of Cornelis Antonisz*, Princeton 1990.

The art of medieval Spain AD 500-1200. Catalogue of the exhibition in the Metropolitan museum of art, New york 1993.

Aue, Hartmann von, *Die Klage. Das (zweite) Buechlein aus dem Ambraser Heldenbuch*. Published by Herta Zutt, Berlin 1968.

Avicenna, see Koning.

Ayrton, Michael, *Giovanni Pisano, sculptor*, London 1969.

Bachmann, Kurt, *Die Spielkarte. Ihre Geschichte in 15. Jahrhundert*, Altenburg 1932.

Baetschmann, Oskar and Pascal Griener, *Hans Holbein*, Zwolle 1997.

Baeumker, Clemens, *Des Alfred von Sareshel (Alfredus Anglicus) Schrift De motu cordis*, Muenster 1923. (Beiträge zur Geschichte der Philosophie des Mittelalters 23).

Balme, see Aristotle, *De partibus*.

Balty, Janine, *Mosaiques antiques de Syrie*, Brussels 1977.

Bange, Petronella, *Spiegels der Christenen. Zelfreflectie en ideaalbeeld in laatmiddeleeuwse moralistisch-didactische traktaten*, Nijmegen 1986. (Middeleeuwse studies 2).

Barberino, F., *Documenti d'amore di Francesco da Barberino*. Edited by F. Egidi, Rome 1905-1927. Societa filologica Romana. (Documenti di storia letteraria 3-6).

Bargellesi, Giacomo, *Palazzo Schifanoia. Gli affreschi nel 'Salone dei mesi' in Ferrara*, Bergamo 1945.

Bargheer, Ernst, *Eingeweide. Lebes- und Seelenkraefte des Leibesinneren im Deutschen Glauben und Brauch*, Berlin Leipzig 1931.

Barnet, Peter (ed.), *Images in ivory. Precious objects of the gothic age*, Detroit 1997. Catalogue of the exhibition at the Detroit institute of arts and the Walters art gallery.

Bartsch, A., *Le peintre graveur*, 21 vols, Vienna 1803-1821, 3.

Belloni, Luigi, *Gli schemi anatomici trecenteschi del codice Trivulziano 836*, Rivista di storia della scienze mediche e naturali 41, 1950, 193-207.

Bendersky, Gordon, *The Olmec heart effigy: earliest image of the human heart*, Perspective in biology and medicine 40, 1997, 348-361.

Benson, Elizabeth P. and Elizabeth H. Boone ed., *Ritual human sacrifice in Mesoamerica*, Washington, 1983. Dumbarton Oaks conference 1979.

Berengario da Carpi, Jacopo, *A short introduction to anatomy (Isagogae breves)*. Translated with an introduction by L.R. Lind, Chicago 1959.

Bianchi, Lidia and Diega Giunta, *Iconografia di S. Caterina da Siena*, Rome 1988.

Bietenholz, Doris, *How comes this means love? A study of the origin of the symbol of love*, Saskatoon 1995.

Bibliotheca Sanctorum. Edited by F. Caraffa et al., 13 vols, Rome 1956, 1.

Bing, Peter and Rip Cohen, *Games of Venus. An anthology of Greek and Roman erotic verse from Sappho to Ovid*, New York, 1991.

Birkhan, Helmut, *Die alchemistische Lehrdichtung des Gratheus filius philosophi in Cod. Vind. 2372*, 2 vols, Vienna 1992.

Blankman, M., *Euterpe's organ. Aspects of Spieghel's* Hart-Spieghel *in interdisciplinary perspective*, in: *From revolt to riches. Culture and history of the Low countries, 1500-1700.* Edited by Theo Hermans and Reinier Salverda, London 1993, 182-195.

Blockbuecher des Mittelalters. Bilderfolgen als Lektuere. Edited by Sabine Mertens and Cornelia Schneider, Mainz 1991. Catalogue of an exhibition in the Gutenberg museum, Mainz.

Boas, M., *De illustratie der Tabula Cebetis*, Het boek 9, 1920, 1-16 and 105-114.

Boeckler, Albert, *Deutsche Buchmalerei vorgotischer Zeit*, Koenigstein 1952.

Bos, A., *La chirurgie de maitre Henri de Mondeville. Traduction contemporaine de l'auteur*, 2 vols, Paris 1897-1898, 1.

Bourguet, Pierre du, *Catalogue des etoffes coptes. Musee national du Louvre*, Paris 1964, 1.

Brijder, H.A.G., *Simply decorated black Siana cups by the Taras painter and Casselcups*, Babesch, 67, 1992, 129-145.

Briquet, C.M., *Les filigranes. Dictionnaire historique des marques du papier des leur apparition vers 1282 jusqu'en 1600*, 4 vols, Amsterdam 1968, 3.

Brown, J. Wood, *The Dominican church of Santa Maria Novella at Florence*, Edinburgh 1902.

Die Brueder Wierix. Graphik in Antwerpen zwischen Bruegel und Rubens. Exhibition catalogue by Christiane Wiebel, Coburg 1995. Kunstsammlungen der Veste Coburg.

Brunner, Hellmut, *Das Herz im aegyptischen Glauben. Das hoerende Herz*, Freiburg Goettingen 1988.

Buhagiar, Mario, *Late Roman and Byzantine catacombs and related burial places in the Maltese islands*, Oxford 1986. (BAR international series 302).

Buisman, J.F., *De ethische denkbeelden van Hendrik Laurensz. Spiegel*, Wageningen 1935.

Burnaby, John, *Amor Dei. A study of the religion of St. Augustin*, London 1938.

Bylebyl, J.J. and Walter Pagel, *The chequered career of Galen's doctrine on the pulmonary veins*, Medical history 15, 1971, 211-229.

Callimachus and Lycophron. With an English translation by A.W. Mair, London 1921. (The Loeb classical library 129).

Camerarius, Joachim, *Symbola et emblemata* (Nueremberg 1590 bis 1604). Facsimile reprint with an introduction by Wolfgang

Harms and Ulla-Britta Kuechen, 2 vols, Graz 1986-1988.

Camille, Michael, *The medieval art of love*, London 1998.

Casserio, Giulio, *De vocis auditusque organis historia anatomica*, Ferrara 1601.

Cats, J., *Proteus ofte minnebeelden verandert in sinnebeelden*, Amsterdam 1658, first edition 1618.

Cebetis Tabula, see Fitzgerald, see also *Cebetis (...) tafereel*, in: Spiegel 1615.

Charbonneau-Lassay, L., *Le bestiaire du Christ. La mysterieuse emblematique du Jesus-Christ*, Bruges 1940.

Chauliac, Guy de, *Chirurgia magna Guidonis de Gauliaco*, Darmstadt 1976.

Chauliac, Guy de, *La grande chirurgie de G. de Chauliac, chirurgien, maistre en medicine de l'universite de Montpellier (1363)*. Translated by E. Nicaise, Paris 1890.

Chauliac, Guy de, see also Wallner

Cheles, Luciano, *The studiolo of Urbino*, Wiesbaden 1986.

Chen Menglei, Jiang Tingxi et al., *Gujin tushu jicheng*, Shanghai 1885-1888.

Choulant, Ludwig, *History and bibliography of anatomic illustration*. Translated and annotated by Mortimer Frank, New York 1962.

Cicero, M. Tullius, *De natura deorum*. With an English translation by H. Rackham, London Cambridge, Mass. 1979. (The Loeb classical library 268).

Clark, Kenneth, *The drawings of Leonardo da Vinci in the collection of her majesty the Queen at Windsor Castle*. 3 vols, London 1969, 3.

Coe, Michael D. (ed.), *The Olmec world. Ritual and rulership*. With essays by Michael D. Coe et al., Princeton 1995. Exhibition catalogue the Art museum, Princeton university, Houston museum of fine arts.

Cohn, W., *Anatomie in China*, Deutsche medizinische Wochenschrift 25, 1899, 496-497.

Colonna, Francesco, *Le songe de Poliphile. Traduction de l'Hypnerotomachia Poliphili*, par Jean Martin. Published and edited by Gilles Polizzi, Paris 1994.

Coornhert, Dirck, *Recht ghebruyck ende misbruyck van tydlicke have*, Amsterdam 1620, first edition 1585.

Coornhert, Dieryck Volckertsz, *Werken*, Amsterdam 1630.

Coornhert, Dirck, *Zedekunst, dat is wellevenskunste vermids waarheyds kennisse vanden mensche van de zonden ende vanden duegden*, 1586.

Corner, G.W., *Anatomical texts of the earlier middle ages. A study in the transmission of culture. With a revised Latin text of* Anatomia Cophonis, Washington 1927.

Corrozet, Gilles, *Hecatomgraphie, Paris 1540*. Preface et notes critiques de Ch. Oulmont, Paris 1905.

Courcelle, Jeanne and Pierre, *Iconographie de Saint Augustin. Les cycles du 14e siecle*, Paris 1965, 1. (Etudes augustiniennes).

Davies, H.W., *Devices of the early printers 1457-1560. Their history and development*, London 1935.

Decouflé, Pierre, *La notion d'ex-voto anatomique chez les Etrusco-Romains. Analyse et synthese*, Brussels 1964. (Collection Latomus 72).

Deichgraeber, Karl, *Hippokrates ueber Entstehung und Aufbau des menschlichen Koerpers*, Leipzig Berlin 1935.

Depuydt, Leo, *Catalogue of coptic manuscripts in the Pierpont Morgan library*, Louvain 1993.

Didron, Victor, *La Charite*, Annales archeologiques 21, 1861, 4-17, 57-66.

Dietz, A., *Das Bild des Herzens*, Fortschritte der Medizin, 109, 1991, 79-82.

Dis, L.M. van and B.H. Erne, *De spelen van zinne vertoond op het landjuweel te Gent van 12-23 juni 1539*, Groningen Batavia 1939.

Dondelinger, Edmund, *Das Totenbuch des Schreibers Ani*, Graz 1978.

Dryander, Joannes, *Anatomia Mundini ad mss. codd. fidem collata* per Ioa. Dryandrum, Marburg [1540].

Ebel, Julia G., *The Family of love: sources of its history in England*, Huntington library quarterly 30, 1966-1967, 331-343.

Edwards, Robert, *The poetry of Guido Guinizelli*, New York London 1987.

Egidi, F., *Le miniature dei Codici Barberini dei 'Documenti d'amore'*, L'arte, 5, 1902, 1-20 and 78-95.

Eijk, Philip J. van der, *Hart en hersenen, bloed en pneuma*, Gewina 18, 1995, 214-229.

Ertzdorff, Xenja von, *Studien zum Begriff des Herzens und seiner Verwendung als Aussagemotiv in der hoefischen Liebeslyrik des 12. Jahrhunderts*, Freiburg i.B. 1958.

Eschmann, Ernst Wilhelm, *Das Herz in Kult und Glauben*, in: Karl Thomae, *Das Herz im Umkreis des Glaubens*, Biberach 1965, 9-50.

Essling, Prince d', *Les livre a figures venetiens de la fin du XVe siecle et du commencement du XVIe*, Florence Paris 1907.

Ettlinger, Leopold D., *Antonio and Piero Pollaiuolo. Complete edition with a critical catalogue*, Oxford 1978.

Eustachius, Bartholomaeus, *Tabulae anatomicae*. First publication by Io.M. Lancisius, Rome 1714. Reprint of the first edition, Holzer 1977.

Fitzgerald, John T. and L. Michael White ed., *The tabula of Cebes. Kebetos pinax*, Chico 1983.

Flinders Petrie, W.M., *Amulets*, London 1914.

Flint, H.L., *The heart. Old and new views*, London 1921.

Fontaine Verwey, H. de la, *Uit de wereld van het boek*. 4 vols, Amsterdam 1975-1997, 1 (1976) *Humanisten, dwepers en rebellen in de zestiende eeuw*, 85-111.

Forrer, R., *Die Graeber und Textilfunde von Achmim-Panopolis*, Strasburg 1891.

Forrer, R; Die fruehchristlichen Altertuemer aus dem Graeberfelde von Achmim-Panopolis, Strassburg 1893

Frank, M., *Manuscript anatomic illustration of the pre-Vesalian period*, in: Choulant, 83-85.

Frantzius, see Aristotle.

Freyhan, R., *The evolution of the Caritas figure in the thirteenth and fourteenth centuries*, Journal of the Warburg and Courtauld institutes 11, 1948, 68-86.

Fruehe Anatomie. Eine Anthologie von Mondino bis Malpighi. Edited by Robert Herrlinger und Fridolf Kudlein, Stuttgart 1967.

Furmerius, Bernardus, *De rerum usu et abusu*, Antwerp 1575.

Galen, Claudius, *On anatomical procedures*. Translation of the surviving books, with introduction and notes by Charles Singer, London 1956.

Galen, Claudius, *On anatomical procedures. The later books*. A translation by W.L.H. Duckworth, Cambridge 1962.

Galen, Claudius, *On the usefulness of the parts of the body (De usu partium)*. Translation with an introduction and commentary by Margaret Tallmadge May, Ithaca 1968.

Galen, Claudius, *On the doctrines of Hippocrates and Plato*. Edition, translation and commentary by Philip de Lacy, 3 vols, Berlin 1978-1984.

Galen, Claudius, *Opera omnia*. Published by C.G. Kuehn, 22 vols, Leipzig 1821-1833. (Medicorum Graecorum opera quae exstant omnia 1-20).

Galle, Philip, *Prosopographia s. virtutum, animi, corporis, bonorum externorum, vitiorum, et affectuum variorum delineatio a Corn. Kiliano illustrata*, 1594.

Gladigow, Burkhard, *Anatomia sacra*, in: *Ancient medicine in its socio-cultural context*. Edited by Ph. J. van der Eijk et al., 2 vols, Amsterdam 1995, 2, 345-361.

Goldschmidt, Adolph, *Die Elfenbeinskulpturen aus der romanischen Zeit XI. bis XII. Jahrhundert*, Berlin 1926.

Gombrich, E.H., *Symbolic images. Studies in the art of the renaissance*, London 1972.

Goss, Charles Mayo, *On anatomy of veins and arteries by Galen of Pergamos*, Anatomical record 141, 1961, 355-366.

Goss, Charles Mayo, *On the anatomy of the uterus*, Anatomical record 144, 1962, 77-84.

Gray's anatomy. The anatomical basis of medicine and surgery, 38th edition, New York 1995. Original title: *Anatomy, descriptive and surgical*, 1858.

The Greek anthology. With an English translation by W.R. Paton, London New York 1916-1918. (The Loeb classical library 67-68, 84-86).

Greve, H.E., *De bronnen van Carel van Mander van 'Het leven der doorluchtighe Nederlandsche en hoogduytsche schilders'*, The Hague 1903. (Quellenstudien zur Hollaendischen Kunstgeschichte 2).

Grimm, Heinrich, *Deutsche Buchdruckersignete des 16. Jahrhunderts. Geschichte, Sinngehalt und Gestaltung kleiner Kulturdokumente*, Wiesbaden 1965.

Gurrieri, Francesco, *Disegni nei manoscritti laurenziani sec. X-XVII*. Catalogue of an exhibition in the Bibliotheca laurenziana, Florence 1979.

Haeften, Benedictus van, *Schola cordis sive aversi a Deo cordis*, Antwerp 1629.

Haetzlerin, Clara, *Liederbuch. Aus der Handschrift des Boehmischen Museums zu Prag*. Published by Carl Haltaus, Leipzig 1840.

Hagen, Victor Wolfgang von, *Het raadsel der verzonken beschavingen van Amerika. Azteken, Maya's, Inca's*, The Hague 1962.

Hahn-Woernle, Birgit, *Die Ebstorfer Weltkarte*, Ebstorf 1987.

Hall, James, *Dictionary of subjects and symbols in art*, London 1974.

Haneveld, G.T., *Het mirakel van het hart*, Baarn 1991. (Bronnen van de Europese cultuur 8).

Harris, C.R.S., *The heart and the vascular system in ancient Greek medicine. From Alcmaeon to Galen*, Oxford 1973.

Harvey, P.D.A., *Mappa mundi. The Hereford world map*, London 1996.

Heckscher, W.S., *Rembrandt's Anatomy of Dr. Nicolaas Tulp. An iconological study*, New York 1958.

Heinrich der Loewe und seine Zeit. Herrschaft und Repraesentation der Welfen 1125-1235. Katalog der Ausstellung, Braunschweig 1995. Published by Jochen Luckhardt und Franz Niehoff, 3 vols, Munich 1995, 1.

Henkel, Arthur and Albrecht Schoene, *Emblemata. Handbuch zur Sinnbildkunst des XVI. und XVII. Jahrhunderts*, Stuttgart 1978.

Hermann, Alfred, *Das steinharte Herz*, Jahrbuch fuer Antike und Christentum 4, 1961, 77-107.

Hill, Boyd H., *Another member of the Sudhoff Fuenfbilderserie - Wellcome ms. 5000*, Sudhoffs Archiv, Vierteljahrsschrift fuer Geschichte der Medizin und der Naturwissenschaften 43, 1959, 13-19.

Hill, Boyd H., *The grain and the spirit in medieval anatomy*, Speculum 40, 1965, 63-73.

Himmel, Hoelle, Fegefeuer. Das Jenzeits im Mittelalter. Catalogue by Peter Jezler. Contributions by Hans-Dietrich Altendorf et al., Zurich Munich 1994. Exhibition in the Schweizerisches Landesmuseum, Zurich and the Wallraf-Richartz-museum, Cologne.

Hippocrates, *Fleshes*. Edited and translated by Paul Potter, Cambridge Mass. London 1995, 8, 127-165.

Hippocrates, *Saemmtliche Werke*. Translated with a commentary by R. Fuchs, Munich 1895-1900.

Hippocratic writings. Edited by G.E.R. Lloyd. Translated by J. Chadwick et al., Harmondsworth, 1983.

Hirschmann, Otto, *Beitrag zu einem Kommentar van Karel van Manders Grondt der edel vrij schilderconst*, Oud Holland 33, 1915, 81-86.

Hitchcock, J., *A confession of the Family of love*, Bulletin of the Institute for historical research 43, 1970, 85-86.

Hoecker, R., *Das Lehrgedicht des Karel van Mander. Text, Uebersetzung und Kommentar nebst Anhang ueber Manders Geschichtskonstruktion und Kunsttheorie*, The Hague 1916.

Hofmann, M., *Ueber die Entwicklung der Lehre vom Bau und den Funktionen des Herzens vom Altertum bis auf Harvey*, Wuerzburg 1913.

Hohenemser, Herbert, *Pulcinella, Harlekin, Hanswurst. Ein Versuch ueber den zeitbestaendigen Typus des Narren auf der Buehne*, Emsdetten 1940.

Hollstein, F.W.H., *Dutch and Flemish etchings, engravings and woodcuts ca. 1450-1700,* Amsterdam.

Hooft, P.C., *Emblemata amatoria*. Published by K. Porteman, Leyden 1983.

Hortus deliciarum. Le 'jardin des delices' de Herrade de Landsberg. Un ms.

alsacien du XIIe siecle. Introduction by El. Rott and J.G. Rott, Strassburg 1945.

Houwaert, Jean Baptista, *Sommare beschrijvinghe vande triumphelijcke incomst*, Antwerp 1579.

Hundt, Magnus, *Antropologium de hominis dignitate, natura, et proprietatibus*, Leipzig 1501.

Israel, Jonathan, *The Dutch republic. Its rise, greatness, and fall, 1477-1806*, Oxford 1998. (Oxford history of early modern Europe).

Jakobi, Christine, *Buchmalerei. Ihre Terminologie in der Kunstgeschichte*, Berlin 1991.

Jansma, N.S.H., *Ornements des manuscripts coptes du monastere Blanc*, Groningen 1973.

Janssen, Han, *De geschiedenis van de speelkaart*, Rijswijk 1985.

Jong, A.C. de, *H.L. Spiegels Hertspiegel 1*, Amsterdam 1930.

Jongh, E.de, *Jan Steen. Dichtbij en toch veraf*, in: Jan Steen. Schilder en verteller, Amsterdam Washington 1996.

Junius, Hadrianus, *Emblemata*. Published by Max Rooses, Antwerp 1902.

Kaftal, George, *St. Catherine in Tuscan painting*, Oxford 1949.

Kaftal, George, *Iconography of the saints in Italian art*, 4 vols, Florence 1952-1986. 1 (1952) *Iconography of the saints in Tuscan painting*. 2 (1986) *Iconography of the saints in Central and South Italian schools of painting*. 3 (1978) *Iconography of the saints in the painting of North East Italy*. With the collaboration of Fabio Bisogni.

Katzenellenbogen, A., *Allegories of the virtues and vices in medieval art. from early Christian times to the thirteenth century*, Toronto Buffalo London 1989.

Kemp-Welch, Alice, *The emblem of St. Ansano*, Burlington magazine 18, 1910-1911, 337-338.

Ketham, Johannes de, *The facsiculus medicinae*. Facsimile of the first (Venetian) edition of 1491. Edited by K. Sudhoff. Introduction by Charles Singer, Milan 1924. (Monumenta medica 2).

Kirschbaum, Engelbert, *Lexikon der christlichen Ikonographie*. With the collaboration of Guenter Bandmann et al., 8 vols, Rome 1994.

Kish, George, *The cosmographic heart: cordiform maps of the 16th century*, Imago mundi 19, 1965, 13-21.

Kleinschmidt, Beda, *Antonius von Padua in Leben und Kunst, Kult und Volkstum*, Duesseldorf 1931.

Knipping, J.B., *De Iconografie van de Contra-reformatie in de Nederlanden*, Hilversum 1939.

197

Knuvelder, G., *Handboek tot de geschiedenis der Nederlandse letterkunde*, 4 vols, 's-Hertogenbosch 1948, 1-2.

Koechlin, Raymond, *Les ivoires gothiques francais*, 3 vols, Paris 1924.

Koenig, Eberhard, *Das liebentbrannte Herz. Der Wiener Codex und der Maler Barthelemy d'Eyck*, Graz 1996.

Koning, P. de, *Trois traites d'anatomie arabes*, Leyden 1903.

Kreytenberg, Gert, *Orcagna's tabernacle in Orsanmichele, Florence*, New York 1994.

Kugler, Hartmut and Eckhard Michael, *Ein Weltbild vor Columbus. Die Ebstorfer Weltkarte*, Weinheim 1991.

Kuhn, Alfred, *Die Illustrationen des Rosenromans*, Jahrbuch der kunsthistorischen Sammlungen des allerhoechsten Kaiserhauses, 31, 1913-1914, 1-66.

Kurth, Betty, *Die deutschen Bildteppiche des Mittelalters*, 3 vols, Vienna 1926.

Laborde, A. de, *Les manuscrits a peintures de la Cite de Dieu de S. Augustine*, Paris 1909.

Ladis, A., *Taddeo Gaddi. Critical appraisal and catalogue raisonne*, Columbia 1982.

Lambert, S.W., *A reading from Andreae Vesalii De corporis humani fabrica liber VII de vivorum sectione nonnula caput XIX*, Bulletin of the New York Academy of medicine 12, 1936, 346-415.

Laske-Fix, Katja, *Der Bildzyklus des Breviari d'amor*, Munich Zurich 1973. (Muenchener kunsthistorische Abhandlungen 5).

Leboucq, G., *Une anatomie antique du coeur humain. Philistion du Locres et le 'Timee' de Platon*, Revue des études grecques 57, 1944, 7-40.

Legner, A., *Romanische Kunst in Deutschland*, Munich 1996.

Lewinsohn, Richard (Morus), *Eine Weltgeschichte des Herzens*, Hamburg 1959.

Leyen, Friedrich von der and Adolf Spater, *Die altdeutschen Wandteppiche im Regensburger Rathaus*, Regensburg 1910.

Liebeschuetz, Hans, *Fulgentius metaforalis*, Leipzig 1926.

Lloyd, see *Hippocratic writings*.

Lonie, I.M., *The paradoxical text 'On the heart'*, Medical history 17, 1973, 1-15 and 137-153.

Luebke, Wilhelm and Max Semrau, *Die Kunst des Mittelalters*, Esslingen 1910.

Lunsingh Scheurleer, Th.H., *Un amphitheatre d'anatomie moralisee*, in: *Leiden university in the seventeenth century: an exchange of learning*. Edited by G.H.M. Posthumus Meyjes, Leyden 1975, 216-277.

Luzuic, S., *Cor Deo devotium Jesu pacifici Salomonis thronus regius*, Antwerp 1628.

Lyna, Frederic, *Le mortifiement de vaine plaisance de Rene d'Anjou. Etude de texte et des manuscripts a peintures*, Brussels Paris 1926.

MacKinney, L.C., *The beginning of western scientific anatomy: new evidence and a revision in interpretation of Mondeville's role*, Medical history 6, 1962, 233-239.

Macrobius, *The Saturnalia*. Translated by Percival Vaughan Davies, New York London 1969. (Records of civilization. Sources and studies 79).

Mâle, Emile, *The gothic image. Religious art in France of the thirteenth century*, New York 1972.

Mancinelli, Fabrizio, *I dipinti della Pinacoteca Vaticana (dall'XI al XV secolo)*, Milan 1992.

Mander, Carel van, *(Schilder-Boeck). Het Leven der oude antijcke doorluchtighe schilders*, Alkmaar 1603 (1604). See also Miedema 1994.

Mander, Karel van, *Den Grondt der edel vry schilder const*, Alkmaar 1603. See also Miedema 1973.

Mannich, Johann, *Sacra emblemata LXXVI in quibus summa uniuscuiusque evangelii rotunde adumbratur*, Nueremberg 1625.

Marchello-Nizia, see *Roman de la poire*.

Margarita Philosophica, see Reisch.

Marle, Raimond van, *Iconographie de l'art profane au moyen-age et à la renaissance*, 2 vols, The Hague 1932.

Mayer, A.L., *Die Sammlung F.H. in Munich*, Pantheon 5, 1930, 263.

McGee, Julie, *Cornelis Corneliszoon van Haarlem (1568-1638)*, Nieuwkoop 1991.

Medicina antiqua. Codex Vindobonensis 93 der Oesterreichischen Nationalbibliothek. Commentary by Hans Zotter, Graz 1996. (Geschichte der Buchkunst 6).

Meer, L.B. van der, *Jecur placentinum and the orientation of the Etruscan haruspex*, Babesch 54, 1979, 49-64.

Meiss, Millard, *The Limbourgs and their contemporaries*, 2 vols, London 1974, 2.

Meiss, Millard, *Painting in Florence and Siena after the black death*, Princeton 1978.

Merindol, C. de, *Le roy Rene et la seconde maison d'Anjou*, Paris 1987.

Mesue, see Pagel.

Middeldorf, U., *Sculptures from the Samuel H. Kress collection, European schools XIV-XIX centuries*, London 1976.

Miedema, Hessel, *Karel van Mander. Den grondt der edel vry schilder-const*, Utrecht 1973.

Miedema, Hessel, *Karel van Mander. The lives of the illustrious Netherlandish and German painters*, Doornspijk 1994.

Minderaa, P., *Twee Hertspiegel problemen*, De nieuwe taalgids, special issue 46, 1953, 79-85.

Moe, Emile van, *Les ethiques, politiques et economiques d'Aristote*, Les tresors des bibliotheques de France 3, 1930, 3-15.

Mondeville, Henry de, *Die Anatomie des Heinrich von Mondeville. Nach einer Handschrift der koeniglichen Bibliothek zu Berlin vom Jahre 1304*. Published by J.L. Pagel, Berlin 1889.

Mondeville, see also Bos.

Montenay, Georgette de, *Monumenta emblematum christianorum virtutum*, Lyon 1571.

Mortimer, Frank, *Manuscript anatomic illustration of the pre-Vesalian period*, in: Choulant, 49-122.

Morus, see Lewinsohn.

Moss, Jean Dietz, *Additional light on the Family of love*, Bulletin of the institute for historical research 47, 1974, 103-105.

Moss, Jean Dietz, *Godded with God: Hendrik Niclaes and his Family of love*, Transactions of the American philosophical society 71, 1981, 8.

Muehsam, Erich, *Zur Lehre vom Bau und der Bedeutung des menschlichen Herzens im klassischen Altertum*, Janus 15, 1910, 797-833.

Muenz, Ludwig, *Bruegel. The drawings*, London New York 1968.

Mundinus, see Adelphus, see also Wickersheimer.

Musa, Mark, *Dante's Vita nuova*, Bloomington London 1973.

Nebel, Werner, *Zur Geschichte der Herzdarstellung*, Archiv fuer Geschichte der Medizin, 28, 1935, 279-295.

Nicaise, see Chauliac.

Niklaus Manuel Deutsch. Maler, Dichter, Staatsmann. Edited by Franz Baechtiger et al., Berne 1979. Catalogue of the exhibition in the Berner Kunstmuseum.

Nisard, Ch., *Histoire des livres populaires, ou de la littérature du colportage*, 2 vols, Paris 1854, 2.

Nijhoff, W., *Nederlandsche houtsneden 1500-1550*, The Hague 1931-1939.

Noot, Jan van der, *The Olympia epics. A facsimile edition of 'Das Buch Extasis', 'Een cort begryp der XII. boecken Olympiados' and 'Abrege des douze livres Olympiades'*. Edited by C.A. Zaalberg, Assen 1956.

Oresme, Nicole, *Le livre de ethiques d'Aristote [traduit par] Nicole Oresme*. With a critical introduction and notes by A.D. Menut, New York 1940.

Orlandi, Stefano and Isuardo P. Grossi, *Santa Maria Novella e i suoi chiostri monumentali. Guida storico artistica*, Florence 1974.

Ovid, *Amores, Ars amatoria*. Edited by E.J. Kenney, Oxford 1994.

Paaw, Pieter, see Vesalius.

Pagel, J.L., *Die angebliche Chirurgie des Johannes Mesue jun.*, Berlin 1893.

Pagel, J.L., see Mondeville.

Pallucchini, Rodolfo, *La pittura Veneziana del trecento*, Venice Rome 1964.

Panofsky, E., *Blind cupid*, in: *Studies in iconology*, New York Evanston 1962, 95-128.

Die Parler und der schoene Stil 1350-1400. Europaeische Kunst unter den Luxemburgern. Published by Anton Legner, 3 vols, Cologne 1978.

Partsch, Suzanna, *Profane Buchmalerei der buergerlichen Gesellschaft im spaet-mittelalterlichen Florenz*, Heidelberg 1980.

Peck, see Aristotle, *History of animals* and *Parts of animals*.

Pellegrino, Francois del, *Le livre de la cure des maladies des yeux de Jean Mesue, medecin arabe du XIe siecle*, Bordeaux 1901.

Perriere, Guillaume de la, *La morosophie*, Lyon 1553.

Perriere, Guillaume de la, *Le theatre des bons engins*, Paris 1539.

Perry, Mary Phillips, *On the psychostasis in christian art*, Burlington magazine 22, 1912-1913, 94-105.

Petrarch, *Lyric poems. The 'Rime sparse' and other lyrics*. Translated and edited by Robert M. Durling, Cambridge London 1976.

Peyligk, Johannes, *Philosophia naturalis compendium*, Leipzig 1499.

Piankoff, Alexander, *Le 'coeur' dans les textes egyptiens depuis l'ancient jusqu'au nouvel empire*, Paris 1930.

Piccard, Gerhard, *Wasserzeichen. Blatt. Blume. Baum*, Stuttgart 1982.

Pilcher, Lewis S., *The Mondino myth*, Medical library and historical journal 4, 1906, 311-331.

Plato, *The Republic*. With an English translation by Paul Shorey. 2 vols, London 1946. (The Loeb classical library 237, 276).

Plutarch, *Moralia 351-384: Isis and Osiris*. Translated by F. Cole Babbitt, 16 vols, London Cambridge, Mass. 1927-1969, 5, 3-191. (The Loeb classical library).

Poeschke, Joachim, *Die Kirche San Francesco in Assisi und ihre Wandmalerein*, Munich 1985.

Poot, Hubert Korneliszoon, *Het groot natuur- en zedekundigh werelttoneel*, Delft 1726-1750.

Pope-Hennesy, John, *Italian gothic sculpture*, London New York 1972.

Pope-Hennesy, John, *Donatello sculptor*, New York London Paris 1993.

Potter, see Hippocrates.

Previtali, A., *Giotto e la sua bottega*, Milan 1993.

Prinsen, J., *Eenige brieven van professor Pieter Pauw aan Orlers*, Oud Holland 23, 1905, 167-174.

Regensburger Buchmalerei. Von fruehkarolingischer Zeit bis zum Ausgang des Mittelalters, Munich 1987.

Regnault, Felix, *Les ex-voto polysplanchniques de l'antiquite*, Bulletin de la Societe francaise d'histoire de la medecine 20, 1926, 135-150.

Reisch, Gregor, *Margarita philosophica*. With an introduction by Lutz Geldsetzer, Duesseldorf 1973. Original edition 1503.

Rene of Anjou, see Lyna, see also Trenkler.

Renner, Dorothee, *Die koptischen Textilien in den vatikanischen Museen*, Wiesbaden 1982.

Rieff Anawalt, Patricia, *Memory clothing: costumes associated with Aztec human sacrifice*, in: Benson 1983, 165-193.

Robicsek, Francis and Donald M. Hales, *Maya heart sacrifice: cultural perspective and surgical technique*, in: Benson 1983, 49-90.

Rollenhagen, Gabriel, *Nucleus emblematum*, Arnhem 1611.

Roman de la poire par Tibaut. Published by Christiane Marchello-Nizia, Paris 1984.

Romano, Serena, *Due affreschi del cappellone degli Spagnuoli; problemi iconologici*, Storia dell'arte 28, 1976, 181-213.

Rossi, G.B. de, *La Roma sotterranea cristiana*, Rome 1864.

Rutschowscaya, Marie-Helene, *Tissues coptes*, Paris 1990.

Sabbe, Maurits, *Plantin, the Moretus and their work*, Brussels 1926.

Saunders, J.B., and Charles D. O'Malley, *The illustrations from the works of Andreas Vesalius of Brussels*, Cleveland New York 1950.

Saxl, Fritz, *Allertugenden und Laster Abbildung*, in: Festschrift fuer Julius Schlosser, Zurich Leipzig Vienna 1927, 104-121.

Saxl, Fritz, *A spiritual encyclopedia*, Journal of the Warburg and Courtauld institutes 5, 1942, 82-143.

Schefold, Karl, *Die Griechen und ihre Nachbarn*, Berlin 1985.

Schiller, Gertrud, *Ikonographie der christlichen Kunst*, Guetersloh 1966-1991.

Schleier, R., *Tabula Cebetis*, Berlin 1973.

Schlueter, Lucy L.E., *Niet alleen. Een kunsthistorisch-ethische plaatsbepaling van tuin en huis in het Convivium religiosum van Erasmus*, Amsterdam 1995.

Schott, A., *Historical notes on the iconography of the heart*, Cardiologia 28, 1956, 229-268.

Schouten, J., *Hartsymboliek*, Antiek 7, 1972-1973, 520-526.

Schramm, Albert, *Die Drucke von Anton Sorg in Augsburg*, Leipzig 1921. (Der Bilderschmuck der Fruedrucke 4).

Schuette, Marie and Sigrid Mueller-Christensen, *Das Stickereiwerk*, Tuebingen 1963.

Seebohm, Almuth, *Apokalypse, ars moriendi, medizinische Traktate, Tugend- und Lasterlehre*, Munich 1995. Microfiche edition.

Seidel, Ernst and Karl Sudhoff, *Drie weitere anatomische Fuenfbilderserien aus Abendland und Morgenland*, Archiv fuer Geschichte der Medizin 3, 1910, 165-187.

Sellink, Manfred, *Een teruggevonden Laatste oordeel van Hendrick Goltzius*, Netherlands yearbook for history of art, 42-43, 1991-1992, 145-158.

Sellink, Manfred, *Philips Galle (1537-1612). Engraver and print publisher in Haarlem and Antwerp*, 3 vols, Leyden 1997.

Sensation. Young Britisch artists from the Saatchi collection. With essays by Brooks Adams et al., London 1997.

Shapley, Fern Rusk, *Paintings from the Samuel H. Kress collection. Italian Schools XIII-XVth century*, London 1966.

Siegel, R.E., *Galen's system of physiology and medicine*, Basle New York 1968.

Singer, Charles, *Beginnings of academic practical anatomy*, in: Choulant, 21a-21r.

Singer 1924, see Ketham

Singer, Charles and C. Rabin, *A prelude to modern science*, Cambridge 1946.

Singer, Charles, *A study in early Renaissance anatomy*, in: *Studies in the history and method of science*. Edited by Charles Singer, London 1955, 80-131.

Singer, Charles, *A short history of anatomy and physiology from the Greeks to Harvey*, New York 1957.

Sluijter, Eric J., *Venus, Visus en Pictura*, Netherlands yearbook for history of art, 42-43, 1991-1992, 337-396.

Spalteholz, Werner and Rudolf Spanner, *Handatlas der Anatomie des Menschen*, Amsterdam 1961.

Spiegel, H.L., *Cebetis des thebaenschen philosoophs tafereel*, in: Spiegel 1615.

Spiegel, H.L., *Hart-Spieghel*, Amsterdam 1614.

Spiegel, H.L., *Hart-Spieghel*, Amsterdam 1615.

Spiegel, H.L., *Hart-Spieghel, Verciert met schoone koopere platen*, Amsterdam 1650.

Spiegel, H.L., *Hertspieghel en andere zede-schriften, meest noyt voor dezen gedrukt*. Published by Hendrik Wetstein, Amsterdam 1694.

Spiegel, H.L., *Hertspieghel en andere zedenschriften met verscheidene nooit gedrukte stukken verrijkt, en door aenteekeningen opgeheldert door P. Vlaming*, Amsterdam 1723, later editions 1730 and 1764.

Spiegel, H.L., *Kebes tafereels kort begrip*, in: Spiegel 1615.

Spiegel, H.L., see also Jong, see also Veenstra.

Spigelius, Adrianus, *Opera quae extant omnia*, Amsterdam 1645.

Sucquet, Antoine, *Den wech des eewich levens*, Antwerp 1620.

Sudhoff, Karl, *Abbildungen zur Anatomie des maitre Henri de Mondeville (ca. 1260-ca. 1320)*, Leipzig 1908. (Studien zur Geschichte der Medizin 4).

Sudhoff, Karl, *Abermals eine neue Handschrift der anatomischen Fuenfbilderserie*, Archiv fuer Geschichte der Medizin 3, 1910, 353-368.

Sudhoff, Karl, *Graphische Darstellungen inneren Koerperorgane*, Archiv fur Geschichte der Medizin 7, 1914, 367-377.

Sudhoff, Karl, *Die Oxforder anatomische Fuenfbilderserie des Cod. Ashmol. 399. Weitere Beiträge zur Geschichte der Anatomie im Mittelalter*, 4. Archiv fuer Geschichte der Medizin 7, 1914, 363-366.

Sudhoff, Karl, *Eine Pariser 'Ketham'. Handschrift aus der Zeit Koenig Karls VI. (1380-1422)*, Archiv fuer Geschichte der Medizin 2, 1909, 84-100.

Sudhoff, Karl, *Tradition und Naturbeachtung in den Illustrationen medizinischer Handschriften und Fruehdrucke vornehmlich des 15. Jahrhunderts*, Leipzig 1907. (Studien zur Geschichte der Medizin 1).

Tabula Cebetis, see Fitzgerald, see also *Cebetis (...) tafereel*, in: Spiegel 1615.

The art of medieval Spain AD 500-1200. Catalogue of the exhibition in the Metropolitan museum of art, New York 1993.

Thiel, P.J.J. van, *Spiegel en het orgel van Euterpe: een Hertspiegel probleem*, in: *Album amicorum J.G. van Gelder*. Edited by J. Bruyn et al., The Hague 1973, 312-320.

Trenkler, Ernst, *Das Livre du cuer d'amours espris des Herzogs Rene von Anjou*, Vienna 1946.

Vaeck, Marc van, *De openhertighe herten en J.J. Starters Steeck-boecxken*, Verslagen en mededelingen van de Koninklijke akademie voor Nederlandse taal- en letterkunde, nieuwe reeks, Gent 1993, 1-31.

Vandenbroeck, Paul, *Beeld van de andere, vertoog over het zelf. Over wilden en narren, boeren en bedelaars*, Ministerie van de Vlaamse gemeenschap 1987. Catalogue of an exhibition. Koninklijk museum voor schone kunsten Antwerp.

Veen, Otto van, *Amorum emblemata*, Antwerp 1608.

Veen, Otto van, *Amoris divini emblemata*, Antwerp 1615.

Veenman, Rene, *Arion op de dolfijn en het titelblad van de Hert-spiegel*, Tijdschrift voor Nederlandse taal- en letterkunde 111, 1995, 225-229.

Veenstra, F., *H.L. Spiegel. Hert-spiegel*, Hilversum 1992.

Veith, Ilza, *The yellow emperor's classic of internal medicine*, Berkeley 1949.

Velde, Carl van de, *Frans Floris (1519-1570). Leven en werken*, Brussel 1975.

Veldman, Ilja M., *Goltzius' zintuigen, seizoenen, elementen, planeten en vier tijden van de dag*, Netherlands yearbook for history of art, 42-43, 1991-1992, 307-336.

Veldman, Ilja M., *Maarten van Heemskerck and Dutch humanism in the sixteenth century*, Maarssen 1977.

Veldman, Ilja M., *De wereld van goed en kwaad. Late prenten van Coornhert*, The Hague 1990.

Venturi, Adolfo, *Giovanni Pisano. Sein Leben und sein Werk*, Florence Munich 1927.

Verdier, Philipe, *Des mysteres grecs a l'age baroque. Commentaires a l'Antrum platonicum de J. Saenredam*, in: *Festschrift Ulrich Middeldorf*. Published by Antje Kosegarten and Peter Tigler, Berlin 1968.

Verwey, A., *Hendrick Laurensz. Spieghel*, Groningen The Hague 1919.

Vesalius, Andreas, *Epitome*, Basel 1543. Facsimile edition by L.R. Lind, New York 1949, (Yale Medical Library 21).

Vesalius, Andreas, *De humani corporis fabrica libri septem*, Basle 1543. See also Saunders.

Vesalius, Andreas, *Epitome anatomica*, Leyden 1616.

Vesalius, Andreas, *Epitome anatomica. Opus redivivum cui accessere. Notae ac commentaria P. Paaw Amsteldamensis*, Amsterdam 1633.

Vignau Wilberg-Schuurman, Thea, *Hoofse mime en burgelijke liefde in de prentkunst rond 1500,* Leyden 1983.

Vinken, P.J., *H.L. Spiegel's Antrum platonicum. A contribution to the iconology of the heart,* Oud Holland 75, 1960, 125-142.

Visscher, Roemer, *Sinnepoppen,* Amsterdam 1614. Published by C.L. Brummel, The Hague 1949.

Wallner, Bjoern, *The Middle English translation of Guy de Chauliac's Anatomy,* Lund 1964.

Wallner, Bjoern, *An interpolated Middle English version of the Anatomy of Guy de Chauliac,* Lund 1995, 1.

Wang Honghan, *Yixue yuanshi,* Shanghai 1989.

Warners, J.D.P., *Cebes en H.L. Spiegel,* De nieuwe taalgids 64, 1971, 1-11.

Weinberg, Florence, *Cave,* in: Jean-Charles Seigneuret, *Dictionary of literary themes and motifs,* New York 1988.

Wessel, Klaus, *Die byzantinische Emailkunst vom V. bis XIII. Jahrhundert,* Recklinghausen 1967.

Wessel, Klaus, *Koptische Kunst. Die Spaetantike in Aegypten,* Recklinghausen 1963.

Wickersheimer, Ernest, *Anatomies de Mondino dei Luzzi et de Guido de Vigevano,* Paris 1926.

Widerkehr, Lena, *Jacob Matham Goltzij privignus. Jacob Matham graveur et ses rapports avec Hendrick Goltzius,* Netherlands yearbook for history of art, 42-43, 1991-1992, 219-260.

Wierix, see *Brueder Wierix.*

Wolf, Armin, *Ikonologie der Ebstorfer Weltkarte und politische Situation des Jahres 1239,* in: Kugler, 54-116.

Yates, Frances A., *The emblematic conceit in Giordano Bruno's* Degli eroici furori *and in Elizabethan sonnet sequences,* Journal of the Warburg and Courtauld institutes 6, 1943, 101-121.

Zanker, Paul, *The mask of Socrates,* Berkeley Los Angeles Oxford 1995.

Zijderveld, A., *Een en ander over Spiegel's Hertspiegel,* Tijdschrift der Nederlandse taal- en letterkunde 44, 1925, 220-229.

Zincgref, Iulius Guilielmus, *Emblematum ethico-politicorum centuria,* Heidelberg 1664. Published by Arthur Henkel and Wolfgang Wiemann, Heidelberg 1986.

First edition 1999
Reprinted with revisions, January 2000

Library of Congress Cataloging-in-Publication Data

Vinken, P.J.
The shape of the heart / by Pierre Vinken
p. 208, 15,5 x 21,5 Cm.
Includes bibliographical references.
ISBN 0-444-82987-3 (alk. Paper)
1. Heart---Iconography 2. Heart---Anatomy. 3. Heart---Symbolic aspects. I, Title.
Qm181. V55 1999
611'.12---dc2199-21440
CIP